When Someone Dies

A practical guide to holistic care at the end of life

Hannah Cooke BSc (Hons), MSc (Econ), MSc, RGN, DN, RNT
University of Manchester
School of Nursing, Midwifery and Health Visiting

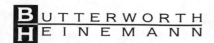

BUTTERWORTH
HEINEMANN

OXFORD AUCKLAND BOSTON JOHANNESBURG MELBOURNE NEW DELHI

Butterworth-Heinemann
Linacre House, Jordan Hill, Oxford OX2 8DP
225 Wildwood Avenue, Woburn, MA 01801-2041
A division of Reed Educational and Professional Publishing Ltd

℞ A member of the Reed Elsevier plc group

First published 2000

© Reed Educational and Professional Publishing Ltd 2000

British Library Cataloguing in Publication Data
A catalogue record for this book is available from the British Library

Library of Congress Cataloguing in Publication Data
A catalogue record for this book is available from the Library of Congress

ISBN 0 7506 4094 4

200696998
09/00

Typeset by Keyword Typesetting Services Ltd, Wallington, Surrey
Printed and bound in Great Britain by Biddles Ltd, Guildford and King's Lynn

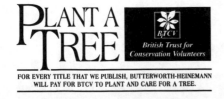

PLANT A TREE

BTCV
British Trust for
Conservation Volunteers

FOR EVERY TITLE THAT WE PUBLISH, BUTTERWORTH-HEINEMANN
WILL PAY FOR BTCV TO PLANT AND CARE FOR A TREE.

This book is dedicated to the memory of Mollie Cooke

Contents

Preface

This book is based on work I did several years ago at Manchester Royal Infirmary providing information and help to staff dealing with dying and bereavement. Staff had a clear idea of the things that they needed to know and I provided information in booklet form. This book has grown from there.

Over several years, while researching and writing this book, I have talked to hundreds of individuals and organizations, including the ones listed in the book. I am extremely grateful to everyone who has shared their thoughts and experiences with me. Special thanks go to the hospital chaplaincy at Manchester Royal Infirmary for their help and support. I must emphasize, however, that any opinions expressed in this book are my own.

I hope you will find this book useful. It has been written primarily for nursing staff but contains much information that other professionals will find helpful. Although I have tried to provide information that will be of immediate use, I hope that above all the book will encourage you to find out more by using the references and resources provided.

Finally, special thanks go to Barbara Henry for typing the final version of the book.

Hannah Cooke

Part One

CARING FOR DYING PATIENTS AND THEIR FAMILIES

Communication with dying patients and their families

1.1 Introduction

The last stages of life should not be seen as defeat, but rather as life's fulfilment. It is not merely a time of negation, but rather an opportunity for positive achievement. One of the ways we can help our patients most is to learn to believe and to expect this. (Saunders 1965)

When a patient will no longer respond to curative treatment and is considered to have a terminal illness, it becomes the responsibility of those who care for him/her to ensure that the patient is helped to live their remaining life as fully as possible. This means that we should use all our available resources to relieve the patient's suffering and promote his/her well being. The patient's time is limited and we must deliver effective, high quality care first time around: we cannot get it right next time.

To ensure death with dignity patients need holistic care. Practical, social, emotional and spiritual needs must be met as well as physical needs. Holistic care demands time, attention and skills from nursing staff and nursing staff must themselves be supported to give this care.

If we wish to enable our dying patients to live until they die we must approach their care in a spirit of partnership, allowing the patients and their families maximum choice and autonomy. Assessing the patient's goals and helping the patient to achieve them is a key feature of good terminal care (Lunt and Jenkins 1983).

1.2 Talking to the dying patient

Talking

Communication in palliative care is important from the moment that the patient first meets a palliative care professional to the last moment of life. (Buckman 1993)

Careful listening is the most important skill in talking to a dying patient. A number of simple guides to *'breaking bad news'* exist and can offer helpful advice (see for example Anstey 1995; Buckman 1984; Buckman 1993;

Fallowfield 1993; Faulkner 1998; Franks 1997; Maguire and Faulkner 1988a, 1988b).

There are some key points to remember when talking to patients with life threatening illness. Some of these may seem obvious but unfortunately there is ample anecdotal and research evidence to suggest that they are often forgotten in the heat of the moment.

Fallowfield (1993) suggests that it is unfortunate that many people are afforded more privacy and consideration in their interview with their bank manager than with health professionals. A quiet and private space is important to any significant conversation. Too often this is difficult to achieve in a busy ward. Offices, treatment rooms or any quiet corner of the ward may have to be used. It is also important that all members of the ward understand the need not to interrupt private conversations with patients. If the conversation has to be conducted at the bedside then closing screens, or sitting close to the patient and talking quietly can help to create privacy.

McLauchlan (1990) gives us the following reminder: 'do not stand holding the door handle like a bus conductor ready to jump off'. It is important not to convey the impression that this is one conversation from which we are longing to escape. Sit down near the patient. Even though you are no doubt busy, try to give the patient the impression that you are prepared to spend some time talking with him/her.

Touch can be comforting and show that you care but some patients will find it intrusive or threatening. Our attitudes to others touching us are influenced by both personal and cultural factors. Touch should be used cautiously and sensitively with an awareness of what is appropriate and of the patient's reactions.

Listening and responding

Many discussions about talking to dying patients focus on the issue of truth telling and the dilemmas that staff experience in deciding what to tell patients about their diagnosis and prognosis. Experienced palliative care professionals tell us that the issue is not *'to tell or not to tell'* but how to listen to what the patient is telling us. If we listen carefully to patients they will usually tell us how much they know and how much they want to know. Research has shown that the majority of dying patients are aware of their prognosis even when they have not been explicitly told (Hinton 1991; McIntosh 1976). If in doubt, we can ask the patient how much they want to be told.

Thus, careful listening is the most important skill when talking to the dying patient. It is a skill that health professionals sometimes lack. It may seem obvious, but the most basic rule is to allow the patient to talk without talking over them or interrupting. Wait for the patient to finish before you start your next sentence. According to Buckman (1993) this, the simplest rule, is the one that is most often ignored.

It is also important to give encouragement and demonstrate that you are attending to what the patient is saying. Do not always fill silences, allow the patient time to think. Show that you have heard what the patient has said by incorporating one or two key phrases that they have used into your responses. Do not repeat the patient's words parrot fashion, however, for you will seem insincere and may irritate the patient (Anstey 1995).

Buckman (1993) says that you must respond to any strong emotions that the patient expresses, for example, rage or grief. If you ignore these you will invalidate what the patient is feeling; the patient may well feel that you are unsympathetic and that it is pointless to confide in you. Respond in a way that shows that such emotions are acceptable unless, of course, the patient is showing inappropriate and threatening behaviour, in which case you should seek support as quickly as possible. In most cases though, it is helpful to show that you understand. Try to identify the cause of the patient's anger or sadness so that you can, if possible, jointly work out an action plan for dealing with what is troubling them. However, Buckman (1993) helpfully advises us of the need to distinguish the '*fixable*' from the '*unfixable*'. Sadly, for some of our patients, we cannot undo the misery of a lifetime in the last few days or weeks of life.

Telling

When imparting information to patients it is important to check what they know about their illness first. Many research studies have demonstrated that lay concepts of health are rather different to medical concepts (Helman 1994). Furthermore other studies have shown that the general public have a hazy and often inaccurate understanding of anatomy and physiology. Patients may have no idea, for example, of the location of their kidneys, what they are for and how big they are (Blackmore 1989).

Try to start from where the patient is now in terms of understanding. Medical information is hard enough to digest at the best of times and more so if the information is threatening. You may remember being in a job interview where, at the end of the interview, the employer asks if you have any questions. You find that your mind is a complete blank. This is how the patient may feel.

Give information in small amounts and check regularly for comprehension. Use plain English, avoid euphemisms and medical jargon. Reinforce information by repeating it or writing it down. A helpful aid is to tape the conversation and allow the patient to take the tape home to replay. Finally, always allow patients time to ask questions and offer them the chance to come back with more questions when the information has sunk in and they have had time to reflect on exactly what they want to know.

Planning

Brewin (1991) suggests that however grave the patient's prognosis, it is important to maintain hope and to suggest something positive that can be done. When making a treatment plan for the patient it is important to elicit the patient's priorities and concerns. Buckman (1993) describes this as the patient's '*shopping list*'. This list may include relief from specific symptoms, preference for place of death, survival for a particular milestone such as a family wedding. There may also be things that patients still want to do before they die. For patients, short term goals are just as important as long term goals. Above all they impart a sense of control and a feeling that the life that is left can still be meaningful to them.

1.3 Staff communication

Continuity of care is important for the dying patient and his or her relatives. A named nurse should be allocated to the patient and should, as far as possible, be responsible for giving and receiving all information about the patient and for discussing the patient's care with relatives and other staff. If it is likely that a patient will die in hospital every effort should be made to ensure that the patient is not transferred between wards during their stay. Patients readmitted from home to die should, wherever possible, be readmitted to a familiar ward (Henley 1986).

Patients may ask any member of staff about their prognosis at any time. All staff involved in caring for patients should have up-to-date knowledge about a patient's condition and level of awareness. It should be clearly understood who will be responsible for imparting information to patients and relatives to avoid staff *'passing the buck'* from one to another (Knight and Field 1981). This will be facilitated by a named nurse or 'Key Worker' arrangement.

May (1993) suggests that disclosure of a terminal prognosis is still an area of potential conflict between doctors and nurses. It is important that a nurse is present when a doctor discusses the patient's diagnosis, prognosis and treatment plan. All too often this still does not happen yet much of the nurse's subsequent work with the patient will involve discussing and interpreting what the doctor has said. Failure to involve the nurse may have disruptive consequences for the care of the patient.

Caring for dying patients is emotionally taxing. Staff need to develop a supportive environment in which nurses and others involved in the patient's care feel able to discuss problems and share their feelings. This may be facilitated by ward meetings to discuss individual cases or by a staff support group. Some other professional groups, for example the chaplaincy, may be willing to help to run such a group.

Further information on facilitating staff support can be obtained from The National Association for Staff Support, including helpful guidance on how to set up a staff support group.

This organization also produces a charter for staff support which some trusts are willing to adopt and implement.

National Association for Staff Support
(within the health care services)
9 Caradon Close
Woking
Surrey. GU21 3DU
Telephone: 01483 771599

1.4 Communication difficulties

Language barriers

If a patient speaks little or no English it is important to ensure that a competent interpreter is available to discuss the patient's condition and care with the patient and his or her family. Unfortunately this is still difficult for many staff to arrange as interpreting services remain very patchy. Although patients' relatives are often used as interpreters, the patient will need an opportunity to talk to staff privately through an interpreter. The patient may have worries or concerns that they do not wish to discuss in the presence of relatives. Sensitive issues should not be discussed while using relatives as interpreters. I have seen a nurse ask a young woman to explain an enema to her grandfather to her obvious embarrassment; incidents like this should be avoided whenever possible. In particular, using children as interpreters should be avoided.

Most hospitals have a list of interpreters available via the hospital switchboard. In some cases the hospital personnel department may have lists of staff with particular language skills. Many hospitals rely on existing staff with language abilities to interpret for patients as a voluntary extra duty. This can be an unsatisfactory arrangement, particularly where the need for an interpreter is frequent. Some hospitals run paid interpreter or linkworker schemes to provide support to patients whose first language is not English. In some areas, local authorities or local voluntary or community groups may run interpreting schemes particularly in the community. If outside interpreters of any description are used, issues of confidentiality must be borne in mind.

Speech impairment

It is important to remember that patients with speech or communication difficulties usually retain a normal awareness of what is going on around them. Every effort must be made to communicate directly with the patient through the use of pencil and paper, language aids etc. Patients with communication difficulties may be particularly aware of tone of voice and non-verbal behaviour and staff need to be sensitive to this in their dealings with them.

- It is important to make sure that you have the patient's full attention and that the patient can see and hear you. Try to eliminate background noise such as the TV.
- Speak slowly and clearly to the patient, but try to speak naturally using normal intonation and phrasing (MacLeod Clark 1985). Try not to sound patronizing. Do not shout.
- Try to use simple sentences.
- Present one idea at a time.
- Repeat what you have said if you are not sure that you have been understood (Easton 1994).

- When asking questions, keep them simple. One question should incorporate one idea, for example: *'Would you like tea?'* not *'Would you like tea, coffee, orange juice or something else?'* Use closed questions which require short or single word answers.
- Give the patient time to answer and listen with full attention however difficult it is to understand. Do not interrupt and never talk about the patient as if he or she is not there.
- If the patient cannot speak try using simple gestures, word cards for yes and no or a word and picture chart. Try a pencil and paper; sometimes people can write what they cannot say.
- Remember that most dysphasic patients are quite as able as you or I to understand what is going on around them.
- Try not to overtire the patient or expect too much from them.
- Look out for signs of fatigue.
- Make use of the speech therapist for advice.
- Find out from relatives what the patient likes and dislikes so that you understand them better as a person.

A Word and Picture Chart is available from the Stroke Association at:

The Stroke Association
CHSA House
Whitecross Street
London. EC1Y 8JJ
Telephone: 0207 490 7999

Visual impairment

Patients with impaired sight may have difficulties with communication when staff do not respond appropriately to their visual impairment. Patients may be unaware of who is talking to them and may be inadequately prepared for a conversation if they have not seen who is approaching them. Patients with recent vision loss may experience particular difficulties.

- When talking to people with poor vision always introduce yourself before you speak. Sit or stand in the position best suited to the patient. Ask the patient where this is.
- Make sure that a person with poor vision knows the position of the call bell, light system and any other important equipment.
- Orientate the patient to the ward, especially the route to the toilet and bathroom. Patients with visual impairment often find it especially hard to find their way back to their own bed. A brightly coloured counterpane can help and you could ask relatives to bring this from home.
- Introduce other staff and especially other patients.
- Always say what you are doing when you are with the patient especially if you are carrying out nursing care.

- Talk clearly but naturally to the patient and always tell the patient when you are leaving. Anyone feels foolish talking to thin air, so remember to spare your patients this embarrassment.

Hearing impairment

If patients are profoundly deaf staff need to assess their preferred method of communication. If patients use British Sign Language, they will need the help of a sign language interpreter. If the patient lip reads, all staff will need instructions on how to communicate with the patient.

For deaf blind patients, information on the deaf blind alphabet and on the finger spelling alphabet can be obtained from the organizations listed in this chapter. (See also Stanley 1995.)

Elderly patients with hearing loss frequently experience loss of high frequencies (for example the consonants 's' and 't'). Speech can become a meaningless jumble and background noise can be particularly detrimental to communication.

- When talking to patients with hearing loss make sure that you are fairly close to the patient on the same level.
- Stand with your face to the light to allow the patient to read your lips. Do not stand with your back to a bright source of light such as a window.
- Cut out background noises by turning off TV, radio etc. (Tolson and McIntosh 1997).
- Speak clearly and slowly using natural speech rhythm. Use simple sentences and do *not* shout.
- If you have not been understood repeat what you have said using different words and phrases.
- Keep still while you are talking, keep your hands away from your face and never talk with your back to the patient.
- Check that any hearing aid is on and working (Tolson 1991).
- Write down any important messages for the patient to keep.
- If the patient has a hearing relative do not talk to the relative and ignore the patient. (See also Salladay and San-Agustin 1984; Taylor and Bishop 1991).

More information about communication difficulties and services available to people with these difficulties can be obtained from the organizations listed below:

> **Action for Dysphasic Adults**
> 1 Royal Street
> London. SE1 7LL
> Telephone: 0207 261 9572

> **Deafblind UK**
> 100 Bridge Street
> Peterborough. PE1 1DY
> Telephone: 01733 358 100

Hearing Concern
(The British Association of the Hard of Hearing)
7/11 Armstrong Road
London. W3 7JL
Telephone: 0208 743 1110
Helpline: 01245 344 600

Henshaw's Society for the Blind
Warwick Road
Manchester. M16
Telephone: 0161 872 1234

Listening Books
12 Lant Street
London. SE1 1QH
Telephone: 0207 407 9417

This organization provides a 'talking book' service to those unable to read due to a disability. Those with a visual handicap should apply to join the RNIB Talking Book Service.

Partially Sighted Society
Sight Centre
9 Plato Place
72–74 St Dionis Road
London. SW6 4TU
Telephone: 0207 371 0289

RNIB
(Royal National Institute for the Blind)
224 Great Portland Street
London. W1N 6AA
Telephone: 0207 388 1266
Helpline: 0345 669 999

Provides support and a wide range of services for anyone with a serious sight problem.

RNIB Talking Book Service
Mount Pleasant
Wembley
Middlesex. 1AO 1RR
Telephone: 0345 626 843

This service provides a library of several thousand recorded books for those unable to read standard print due to a visual impairment.

RNID
(Royal National Institute for the Deaf)
19–23 Featherstone Street
London. EC1X 8SL
Telephone: 0207 296 8000

Talking Newspapers Association of the UK
National Recording Centre
Heathfield
East Sussex. TN21 8DB

Provides national newspapers and magazines on audiotape, computer disc or e-mail for visually impaired or disabled people. A choice of over 200 newspapers and magazines are available. There is a small annual fee.

1.5 Communicating with relatives

The needs of relatives

When a patient is terminally ill his or her relatives will need support, information and counselling. Meeting the needs of relatives can help to promote good communication between the patient and their family, thus improving the patient's psychological well being (Lugton 1987). Support for relatives will also help them to assist in caring for the patient and is particularly important if the patient's discharge home is envisaged (Lugton 1987).

Good communication with relatives can help them to anticipate the patient's death and thus lessen the initial shock of bereavement (Andershed and Ternestedt 1998; Brewin 1996; Penson 1990).

Studies of relatives' views of the support that they received from ward staff has highlighted a number of deficiencies, in particular poor communication (Bond 1982; Hampe 1975; Molter 1979). Surveys of relatives of the dying have also produced information on relatives' own views as to the support they required (Breu and Dracup 1978; Coulter 1988; Hampe 1975; Nash 1988). The following are key points to consider.

Relatives express the need to:

- Be with the dying patient.
- Help to care for the dying patient.
- Be reassured that the dying patient is receiving good professional care.
- Be informed of diagnosis, treatment and prognosis. Information should be regularly updated.
- Discuss and plan care of the patient if the patient is to be discharged.
- Be informed of the patient's impending death if this is thought to be imminent.
- Have comfort and support from other relatives and friends.
- Have opportunities for rest, sleep and facilities for washing and changing, meals and hot drinks.
- Have adequate privacy.
- Receive spiritual support from appropriate chaplains or ministers if required.
- Receive support and acceptance from ward staff.

Contacting relatives

Relatives may wish to be with the patient at the time of death. It is important therefore that an accurate record of the address and contact telephone numbers of next of kin are kept in the patient's notes. Nursing staff should find out who the patient and relatives would wish to be contacted if the patient's condition deteriorates. Relatives should also be asked whether they would wish to be called out during the night. The relatives' wishes should be recorded in the patient's nursing notes.

Supporting relatives

Relatives may need support and guidance in sitting with a dying patient. Relatives should not be left alone for long periods with a dying patient without regular contact from nursing staff, they need to be shown how to use the nurse call system and encouraged to call the nurse whenever they feel the need for reassurance or assistance. It can help to offer to sit with the patient to enable relatives to take meal breaks etc. Arrangements should be made for relatives to have access to facilities for hot drinks and meals. Overnight accommodation may need to be arranged in the hospital if necessary and consideration should be given to enabling the relatives to obtain sleep and rest.

If appropriate, relatives may be encouraged to participate in the care of the patient. If the patient is unresponsive, relatives need to be told that the patient may still be able to hear them and can be encouraged to talk to the patient. Nothing should be said in front of a dying patient which the nurse or relative would not wish them to hear however unresponsive they seem.

Relatives may be anxious about recognizing the moment of death and should be encouraged to call the nursing staff for support if they are worried about any change in the patient's condition. Some relatives may be afraid of missing the moment of death and may be reluctant to leave the bedside. They should be reassured that the patient will not be left alone while they are away but ultimately supported in making their own decision. Relatives who are encouraged to leave the bedside against their own inclinations can suffer a profound sense of guilt afterwards if the patient dies during their absence. For this reason it is also advisable not to exclude relatives when carrying out nursing care.

Relatives need to be given as much privacy as possible and if a side ward is available the patient and his/her relatives should be consulted on whether they wish to use it.

At the time of death and immediately afterwards relatives will benefit from being allowed to stay with the patient for as long as they wish. They should be offered a private area in the ward to sit in after the death and the support of a staff member who is able to discuss the patient's death. Staff should offer to telephone other family and friends if needed.

Sudden deaths

Approximately one-third of patients who die in hospital do so within a few hours of admission (Yates *et al.* 1990). Often this will be as a result of a sudden illness or accident. Nursing and medical efforts will focus on resuscitating the patient but the needs of the patient's family are also important.

A number of studies have highlighted the fact that staff feel inadequately prepared and supported when dealing with the suddenly bereaved (Granger *et al.* 1995; Lloyd-Richards and Rees 1996). A useful report by The British Association of Accident and Emergency Medicine and Royal College of Nursing (1995) gives helpful detailed guidance on the management of sudden death in Accident and Emergency Departments.

Individuals exposed to sudden bereavement have particular problems in coming to terms with their loss as they have had no opportunity to anticipate the event (Lundin 1984; Parkes 1990). Survivors of sudden bereavement often report a strong sense of unreality and may find it difficult to accept their loss, particularly if they have not been allowed to see the deceased (Awooner-Renner 1991). Work with the suddenly bereaved has identified a number of ways in which health care staff can help to support relatives (Cooke 1992; Coolican 1994; Dent *et al.* 1996; Ellison 1992; Finlay and Dallimore 1991; McLauchlan 1990; Wright 1992). The following points should be considered:

- Inform relatives regularly about the patient's condition and progress. Repeated simple explanations using non technical language should be given. Euphemisms should be avoided. Avoid giving false hope.
- Allow access to the critically ill/dying patient during the resuscitation attempt if relatives want this.
- Make a private room available for relatives.
- Allocate specific responsibility to one nurse to liaise with relatives.
- When bad news is being broken, relatives should be informed in private and in an unhurried manner. Time should be allowed for relatives to ask questions. Euphemisms must be avoided. The patient should be described as having died.
- Allow time for relatives to spend with the person who has died. Offer nursing support if required.
- Offer the services of a hospital chaplain.
- Ensure that relatives have transport home and support from friends/relatives over the next 24 hours.
- Inform the family's GP immediately.
- Give relatives a phone number to contact a member of staff in case of further queries after leaving the hospital.
- Give relatives written information on practical arrangements following the death and on support groups in the community.

1.6 Training in counselling and communication

Training in counselling and communication may be available locally from a variety of sources. Your local Further Education College or University Extramural Department may provide counselling courses. Specific courses for nurses may be available from your local Nurse Education Department. Both Cruse and Relate provide counselling training and your local branch will be listed in the telephone directory. There are also specialist centres for counselling training in larger cities. The professional body for counsellors is the British Association of Counselling who can provide lists of accredited courses.

British Association of Counselling
1 Regent Place
Rugby. CV21 2PJ
Telephone: 01788 578328

1.7 Patient education and support organizations

Patients with life threatening illnesses require a lot of emotional, practical and financial support. They also need understandable and unbiased information about their condition. There are many sources of information available to patients nowadays through the media and increasingly through the World Wide Web. Information on the World Wide Web needs to be treated with caution and sources checked. Some websites provide information that is inaccurate and misleading. There are many voluntary and self-help groups providing help and support to the seriously ill. Many produce information literature as well as organizing counselling, support and a range of practical services. Some groups also now have websites. These groups provide the best sources of information and support for your patients. A list of selected organizations is included here with brief details of the services they offer.

Cancer organizations

Call Centre –Cancer Aid and Listening Line
Swan Buildings
20 Swan Street
Manchester. M4 5JW
Telephone: 0161 835 2586

A support group with a 24 hour helpline.

Cancer Bacup
3 Bath Place
Rivington Street
London. EC2A 3JR
Telephone: 0207 696 9003
Helpline: 0800 181 199

Provides information and support by phone and letter. A wide range of information booklets are available free to cancer sufferers and their families, including *Facing the Challenge of Advanced Cancer*. Face to face counselling is available in London and Glasgow.

London: Telephone: 0207 696 9000
Glasgow: Telephone: 0141 553 1553

Cancer Black Care
16 Dalston Lane
London. E8 3AZ
Helpline: 0207 249 1097

Information and advice for black people affected by cancer. Also offers training to health professionals.

Cancer Care Society
Jane Scarth House
39 The Hundred
Romsey
Hants. SO51 8GE
Telephone: 01794 830374

Offers emotional support and counselling by phone. There are also support groups throughout the country.

Cancer Counselling and Education Centre
64 Fleet Street
Hampstead
London. NW3 2QT
Telephone: 0207 482 4296

Cancerlink
11–21 Northdown Street
London. N1 9BN
Telephone: 0207 833 2818
Helpline: 0800 132 905

Asian Cancer Information Line: 0800 590 415
Mac Helpline (for young people): 0800 591 028

Provides support and information by telephone and letter. Supports over 300 self-help groups nationwide. Publishes an annual *Directory of Cancer Support and Self Help Groups*.

Publishes a range of information booklets in English, Hindi, Punjabi, Gujerati, Urdu, Bengali and Chinese. Audio tapes are also available.

E.mail: cancerlink @ canlink.demon.co.uk

Gayscan
50 Avenue Road
London. N12 8PY
Telephone: 01275 847 484

A national group offering mutual help and support to gay people living with cancer.

Hairline International
Lyons Court
1668 High Street
Knowle
West Midlands. B93 OLY
Telephone: 01564 775 281

Gives advice on coping with hair loss.

Irish Cancer Society
5 Northumberland Road
Dublin 4
Ireland
Telephone: 010 353 668 1855

Macmillan Cancer Relief
Anchor House
15/19 Britten Street
London. SW3 3TZ
Telephone: 0207 351 7811
Information Line: 0845 601 6161

Scotland and Northern Ireland office:
9 Castle Terrace
Edinburgh. EH1 2DP
Telephone: 0131 229 3276

Supports and develops cancer services and education within the NHS, i.e.Macmillan nurses. A *Directory of Macmillan Services* is available on request.

Also provides some grants to cancer sufferers. Applications for grants must be made by an appropriate professional. Application forms and details can be obtained from the address above.

Marie Curie Cancer Care
28 Belgrave Square
London. SW1X 8QG
Telephone: 0207 235 3325

Scottish office:
21 Rutland Street
Edinburgh. EH1 2AH
Telephone: 0131 229 8332

Website: www.mariecurie.org.uk

Provides nursing care in eleven inpatient centres and a home nursing service. Education for professionals is also provided.

National Cancer Alliance
PO Box 579
Oxford. OX4 1LP
Telephone: 01865 793566 (09.30–16.30hr)

A voluntary organization formed to voice the concerns and opinions of people affected by cancer. Provides information about good care and what standards of care and treatment people have a right to expect.

Tak Tent
(Cancer support, Scotland)
The Western Infirmary
Block 20, Western Court
100 University Avenue
Glasgow. G12 6SQ
Telephone: 0141 211 1932 (Mon–Fri: 10.00–15.00hr)

Provides practical and emotional support to cancer patients in Scotland. Provides information service and runs local support groups.

The Tenovus Cancer Information Centre
College Buildings
Courtenay Road
Splott
Cardiff. CF1 1SA
Telephone: 0800 526 527 (Mon–Fri: 09.00–17.00hr)

Provides support for cancer patients in Wales and a freephone helpline.

The Ulster Cancer Foundation
40–42 Eglantine Avenue
Belfast. BJ9 6DX
Helpline: 028 90663 439 (09.30–12.30hr)

Support organizations for specific types of cancer

Breast Cancer Care
Kiln House
210 New Kings Road
London. SW6 4NZ
Telephone: 0207 384 2344
Freephone: 0500 245 345

Free help and support for people with cancer and their families.

Brain Tumour Foundation
PO Box 162
New Malden
Surrey. KT3 3YN
Telephone: 0208 336 2020

British Colostomy Association
15 Station Road
Reading
Berkshire. TG1 1LG
Telephone: 0118 939 1537

An information and advisory service for people with colostomies.

Changing Faces
1–2 Junction Mews
London. W2 1PN
Telephone: 0207 706 4232

A national organization for people with facial disfigurement. Their wide ranging information service includes booklets and videos.

I.A. Ileostomy and Internal Pouch Support Group
PO Box 123
Scunthorpe. DN15 9YW

Urostomy Association
Buckland
Beaumont Park
Danbury
Essex. CM3 4DE
Telephone: 01245 224 294

National Association of Laryngectomy Clubs
Ground Floor
6 Rickett Street
London. SW6 1RU
Telephone: 0207 381 9993

Leukaemia Care Society
14 Kingfisher Court
Kenny Bridge
Pinhoe
Exeter. EX4 8JN

Hodgkins Disease and Lymphoma Association
PO Box 275
Haddenham
Aylesbury
Bucks. HP17 8JJ
Telephone: 01844 291 500

Let's Face It
10 Wood End
Crowthorne
Berks. RG11 6DQ

An organization for the facially disfigured.

Lymphoedema Support Network
St. Lukes Crypt
Sydney Street
London. SW3 6NH
Telephone: 0207 351 4480

Provides information on lymphoedema management to patients and healthcare professionals.

Prostate Cancer Society
Du Cane Road
London. W12 0NN
Telephone: 0208 383 1948 (Thurs and Fri am)

Rage (Radiotherapy Action Group Exposure)
24 Edgeborough Way
Bromley
Kent. BR1 2UA
Telephone: 0208 460 7476

Campaigning group for breast cancer patients suffering damage from radiotherapy treatment.

Save Our Sons
(Support for men and boys with testicular cancer)
Shirley Wilcox
Tides Reach
1 Kite Hill
Wooton Bridge
Isle of Wight. PO33 4LA

Information booklets for people with cancer

Both Cancerlink and Bacup provide a good range of patient information booklets. These are free to patients but health professionals may be charged for them.

The Royal Marsden Hospital also provide a series of educational booklets for cancer patients. Prices on application. Enquiries and order to:

Hochland and Hochland Publications Limited
174a Ashley Road
Hale
Cheshire. WA15 9SF

Recommended reading for people with cancer

Chris and Sue Williams (1986) *Cancer : A Guide for Patients and Their Families*. Wiley.
Rachel Clyne (1989) *Cancer, Your Life, Your Choice*. Thorsons.
Carolyn Faulder (1989) *The Women's Cancer Book*. Virago.
Karol Sikora and Hilary Thomas (1989) *Fight Cancer*. BBC Books.
Val Speechley and Maxine Rosenfield (1992) *Cancer Information at Your Fingertips*. Class Publishing.

Declaration of Rights of People with Cancer

The Declaration of Rights of People with Cancer has been produced by representatives of 350 cancer support and self-help groups. It is designed to act as a starting point for debate and to encourage improvements in service provision for people with cancer. Individuals and organizations can pledge their support to the Declaration. Copies are obtainable from Cancerlink.

Organizations for children and young people with life threatening conditions

ACT
(Association for Children with Life Threatening or Terminal Conditions and their Families)
65 St. Michael's Hill
Bristol. BS2 8DZ
Telephone: 0117 922 1556

Cancer and Leukaemia in Childhood (CLIC)
12/13 Kings Square
Bristol. BS2 8JH
Telephone: 0117 924 8844

Contact a Family
170 Tottenham Court Road
London. W1P OHA
Telephone: 0207 383 3555

Christian Lewis Trust
62 Walters Road
Swansea
West Glamorgan
Wales. SA1 4PT
Helpline: 0800 30 30 31

Provides a national helpline for families of children with cancer; also provides care and support.

Help Adolescents With Cancer
151 Moston Lane East
New Moston
Manchester. M40 3GJ
Telephone: 0161 688 6244

A national charity offering support to families where an adolescent has cancer.

The Teenage Cancer Trust
Kirkman House
Kirkman Place
54a Tottenham Court Road
London. W1P 9RF
Telephone: 0207 436 2877

Support for people with AIDS

The Terence Higgins Trust
52–54 Grays Inn Road
London. WC1X 8JU

Telephone: Administration: 0207 831 0330
Helpline: 0207 242 1010 (12.00–22.00 hr)
Legal Line: 0207 405 2381

Provides information and advice by telephone and letter. This includes advice on benefits, housing and a legal line giving advice on wills, insurance and other legal matters. The Trust publishes a range of information leaflets and health promotion materials. Contact Terence Higgins Enterprises Limited at the address above.

The Trust also administers a hardship fund for people with AIDS nationally and provides training and information for professionals caring for people with AIDS.

Body Positive
14 Greek Street
Soho
London. W1V 5LE
Telephone: 0207 287 8010
e.mail: bp@bodypositive.demon.co.uk.

Offers information, advice and support to people with HIV/AIDS. Services include a library and internet lounge, treatment advisory service, counselling, legal advice, welfare advice and a telephone helpline.

Immune Development Trust
90–92 Islington High Street
London. N1 8EG
Telephone: 0207 704 1717 (Client Services)

A charity dedicated to delivering complementary therapies to people with immune related diseases.

ACET (AIDS Care Education and Training)
P.O. Box 3693
London. SW15 2BQ

National AIDS Helplines

Freefone 0800 567 123 (24 hours)

Afro Caribbean 0800 282 445 (Fri: 18.00–22.00 hr)

Arabic 0800 282 447 (Wed: 18.00–22.00 hr)

Cantonese and Mandarin 0800 282 445 (Tues: 18.00–22.00 hr)

Urdu, Hindi, Punjabi Gujerati and Bengali 0800 282 445
(Wed: 18.00–22.00 hr)

Minicom 0800 521 361 (Daily: 10.00–22.00 hr)

Information in braille is available from the RNIB.

Mildmay Mission Hospital
Hackney Road
Bethnal Green
London. E2 7NA
Telephone: 0207 653 6300

A specialist hospice for people with HIV/AIDS. The Hospice Information Service can supply information on other hospices who treat patients with AIDS.

Organizations for people with other life threatening illnesses

The Stroke Association
Stroke House
Whitecross Street
London. EC1Y 8JJ
Telephone: 0207 490 7999

Provides information and advice for people with strokes. Publishes a range of information booklets and videos. Supports a network of local 'Stroke Clubs', runs a volunteer stroke scheme to assist people who have suffered a stroke and their families.

British Lung Foundation
78 Hatton Garden
London. EC1N 8JR
Telephone: 0207 831 5831

For advice and publications on chronic bronchitis, emphysema, bronchiectasis, chronic obstructive airways disease and all other lung diseases.

British Heart Foundation
14 Fitzhardinge Street
London. W1H 4DH
Telephone: 0207 935 0185

For advice and publications on heart disease.

Alzheimers Disease Society
Gordon House
10 Greencoats Place
London. SW1
Telephone: 0207 306 0606
Helpline: 0207 306 0808

Multiple Sclerosis Society
25 Effie Road
Fulham
London. SW6 1EE
Telephone: 0207 610 7171
Helpline: 0207 371 8000

Parkinsons Disease Society
22 Upper Woburn Place
London. WC1H ORA
Telephone: 0207 383 3513
Helpline: 0207 388 5798

Motor Neurone Disease Association
PO Box 246
Northampton. NN1 2PR
Telephone: 01604 250 505
Helpline: 0345 626 262

Useful local addresses (for personal use)

References

Andershed, B. and Ternestedt, B. (1998) 'Involvement of relatives in the care of the dying in different care cultures: involvement in the dark or in the light', *Cancer Nursing* 21(2): 106–16.

Anstey, S. (1995) 'Communication', in Penson J. and Fisher R. (eds) *Palliative Care for People with Cancer*. London: Arnold, pp. 246–9.

Awooner-Renner, S. (1991) 'I desperately needed to see my son', *British Medical Journal* 302: 356.

Blackmore, S. (1989) 'A survey of general medical knowledge among university students : its implications for informed consent and health education', *Senior Nurse* 19(10): 17–20.

Bond, S. (1982) 'Communicating with families of cancer patients', *Nursing Times* 9 (78): 962–5.

Breu, C. and Dracup, K. (1978) 'Helping the spouses of critically ill patients', *American Journal of Nursing* June, pp. 50–3.

Brewin, T. (1991) 'Three ways of giving bad news', *Lancet* 337: 1207–9.

Brewin, T. (1996) *Relating to the Relatives: Breaking Bad News, Communication and Support.* Oxford: Radcliffe Medical Press.

Bridgman, H. and Carr, E. (1998) 'Providing family care in hospital', *Nursing Times* 94(1): 44–7.

British Association for Accident and Emergency Medicine and Royal College of Nursing (1995) *Bereavement Care and A and E Departments.* London: Royal College of Nursing.

Buckman, R. (1984) 'Breaking bad news: why is it still so difficult?', *British Medical Journal* 88(1): 1597–9.

Buckman, R. (1993) 'Communication in palliative care: a practical guide', in Doyle, D. (ed.) *Oxford Textbook of Palliative Medicine*, Section 2.5. Oxford: Oxford University Press, pp. 47–61.

Cooke, M.W. (1992) 'Management of sudden bereavement in the accident and emergency department', *British Medical Journal* 304: 1207–9.

Coolican, M.B. (1994) 'Families: facing the sudden death of a loved one', *Critical Care Nursing Clinics of North America* 6(3): 607–12.

Coulter, M. (1988) 'The needs of family members of patients in intensive care units', *Intensive Care Nursing* 5: 4–10.

Dent, A., Condon, L., Blair, P.P. and Fleming, P.P. (1996) 'A study of bereavement care after a sudden and unexpected death', *Archives of Disease in Childhood* 74(6): 522–6.

Easton, K.L. (1994) 'Distinct probabilities ... things to remember when working with aphasic patients', *Rehabilitation Nursing* 19(5): 303.

Ellison, G. (1992) 'A private disaster', *Nursing Times* 88(52): 59.

Fallowfield, L. (1993) 'Giving sad and bad news', *Lancet* 341: 476–9.

Faulkner, A. (1998) 'ABC of Palliative Care. Communication with patients, families and other professionals', *British Medical Journal* 316: 130–2.

Finlay, I. and Dallimore, D. (1991) 'Your child is dead', *British Medical Journal* 302: 24–5.

Franks, A. (1997) 'Breaking bad news and the challenge of communication', *European Journal of Palliative Care* 4(2): 61–5.

Granger, C.E., George, C. and Shelly, M.P. (1995) 'The management of bereavement in Intensive Care Units', *Intensive Care Medicine* 21(5): 429–36.

Hampe, S.O. (1975) 'Needs of the grieving spouse in the hospital setting', *Nursing Research* 24(2): 113–21.

Henley, A. (1986) *Good Practice in Hospital Care for Dying Patients*. London: Kings Fund.

Helman, C. (1994) *Culture, Health and Illness: An Introduction for Health Professionals*, 3rd edn. Oxford: Butterworth-Heinemann.

Hinton, J. (1991) *Dying*, 2nd edn. Harmondsworth: Penguin.

Knight, M. and Field, D. (1981) 'A silent conspiracy: coping with dying patients in an acute surgical ward', *Journal of Advanced Nursing* 6: 221–9.

Lloyd-Richards, C. and Rees, C. (1996) 'Clinical management: hospital nurses' bereavement support for relatives', *International Journal of Palliative Nursing* 2(2): 106–10.

Lugton, J. (1987) *Communication With Dying Patients and Their Families*. London: Austen Cornish.

Lundin, T. (1984) 'Morbidity following sudden and unexpected bereavement', *British Journal of Psychiatry* 144: 84–8.

Lunt, B. and Jenkins, J. (1983) 'Goal setting in terminal care: a method of recording treatment, aims and priorities', *Journal of Advanced Nursing* 8: 495–505.

MacLeod Clark, J. (1985) 'Communicating with elderly people', in Redfern, A. (ed.) *Nursing Elderly People*. Edinburgh: Churchill Livingstone.

Maguire, P.P. and Faulkner, A. (1988a) 'Communicate with cancer patients: 1 Handling bad news and difficult questions', *British Medical Journal* 297: 907–9.

Maguire, P.P. and Faulkner, A. (1988b) 'Communicate with cancer patients: 2 Handling uncertainty, collusion and denial', *British Medical Journal* 297: 972–5.

May, C. (1993) 'Disclosure of terminal prognosis in a general hospital: the nurse's view', *Journal of Advanced Nursing* 18: 1362–8.

McIntosh, J. (1976) 'Patients' awareness and desire for information about diagnosed but undisclosed malignant disease', *Lancet* ii: 855.

McLauchlan, C. (1990) 'Handling distressed relatives and breaking bad news', *British Medical Journal* 301: 1145–9.

Molter, N.C. (1979) 'Needs of critically ill patients: a descriptive study', *Nursing Research* 8: 2.

Nash, A. (1988) 'The role of the nurse in family support', in Wilson-Barnett, J. and Raiman, J. (eds) *Nursing Issues and Research in Terminal Care*. London: John Wiley.

Parkes, C.M. (1990) 'Risk factors in bereavement: implications for the prevention and treatment of pathology in grief', *Psychiatric Annals* 20(6): 308–13.

Penson, J. (1990) *Bereavement: A Guide for Nurses*. London: Harper and Row.

Salladay, S. and San-Agustin, T. (1984) 'Special needs of the deaf dying patient', *Death Education* 8(4): 257–69.

Saunders, C.M. (1965) 'The last stages of life', *American Journal of Nursing* 65: 70–5.
Stanley, C. (1995) 'The healing touch', *Nursing Times* 91(29): 36–40.
Taylor, G. and Bishop, J. (1991) (eds) *Being Deaf: The Experience of Deafness*. Milton Keynes: Open University Press.
Tolson, D. (1991) 'Making sense of hearing aids', *Nursing Times* 87(18): 36–8.
Tolson, D. and McIntosh, J. (1997) 'Listening in the care environment – chaos or clarity for the hearing impaired elderly person', *International Journal of Nursing Studies* 34(3): 173–82.
Wright, B. (1992) *Sudden Death: Intervention Skills for the Caring Professionals*. London: Longman.
Yates, D. *et al.* (1990) 'Care of the suddenly bereaved', *British Medical Journal* 301: 29–31.

2

Choices for dying people

Patients who are dying should be allowed as much freedom of choice as is practicable regarding how they will spend the life that is left to them. In order to enable the patient to make informed choices it is important that conversations with the dying patient and family are conducted in a spirit of openness. This does not imply brutal frankness but a willingness to listen and to answer questions and address the patient's concerns.

2.1 Choices about treatment and care

The patient who is a fully aware adult has a right to choose whether or not to continue with medical treatment. No other adult has a right to make these decisions for the patient (Faulder 1985). In order to make these choices the patient needs to be fully informed about the treatment options and to understand the possible benefit, risks and potential side effects of treatment. Other important considerations for the patient may be the effect of opting for a course of treatment on their quality of life and on planned activities (Saunders and Brown 1995). Will they have to cancel a much needed holiday? Will they have to spend time as an in-patient and be parted from their family? Patients should be encouraged to voice their concerns so that treatment can be planned to meet their needs and priorities as fully as possible. Things should not be done just because they are the routine treatment in a particular setting such as the hospital. This can apply equally to some hospices, where staff may be reluctant to instigate invasive treatment such as intravenous infusions because it is not their way of doing things.

It is important that nursing care is planned in conjunction with the patient and his or her family. Goal setting should be an activity shared with the patient and their family. Routine nursing interventions such as observations of blood pressure, pulse and temperature should be considered carefully and discontinued if they are no longer required. Patients should be allowed to make their own decisions about their daily routine and level of activity as well as the amount of assistance they require with activities of daily living. The nurse in acute areas is used to getting patients 'up and about' in the interests of rehabilitation. This can be inappropriate for the dying patient who may have different priorities for the use of their limited energies.

Decisions about where to care for the patient need to be made in conjunction with the patient. Some patients may prefer the privacy of a side ward while others will prefer to be part of the life of the ward.

Nursing staff at St Christopher's Hospice have devised a nursing model specifically relating to terminal care. An information pack containing details of the model, assessment sheets and St Christopher's nursing philosophy can be obtained from the study centre at St Christopher's.

The Study Centre
St Christopher's Hospice
51–59 Lawrie Park Road
Sydenham. SE26 6OZ
Telephone: 0208 778 9252

2.2 Choices about where to live and where to die

Many patients may wish to go home to die or spend their last weeks in a hospice (Parkes 1985; Townsend *et al.* 1990). The hospice movement was founded in the UK by Dame Cicely Saunders to improve the care of the dying. Most hospices are charitable institutions outside the NHS. Hospices provide a range of services including inpatient care, day care and care at home. Every effort should be made to arrange for the appropriate care and support to be given to patients and their families. If a patient requires social care an urgent referral under the Community Care Act can be made by contacting the duty social worker. The Macmillan nurses and district nursing staff can also provide support and care to patients and their families at home. In some districts the Marie Curie foundation fund a night nursing service for cancer patients. Some hospices offer day care/out-patient facilities to support patients and their families at home and they may also offer respite and convalescent inpatient care.

Finding home care

Macmillan nurses offer specialist nursing advice and support to cancer patients. Macmillan nurses and district nurses are usually employed by the local community healthcare trust. The Macmillan Cancer Relief National Office may be able to advise concerning the availability of Macmillan nurses in a particular locality and publish the Directory of Macmillan Services. Contact:

Macmillan Cancer Relief
15/19 Britten Street
London. SW3 3TZ
Telephone: 0207 351 7811
Macmillan Information Line: 0845 601 6161

Scotland and Northern Ireland office:
9 Castle Terrace
Edinburgh. EH1 2DP
Telephone: 0131 229 3276

Marie Curie Cancer Care provides 5,000 Marie Curie Nurses throughout the UK who are normally available through the local district nursing services. Marie Curie nurses can also be contacted through the Marie Curie Nurse Managers in each region. Contact:

Marie Curie Cancer Care
Head Office
28 Belgrave Square
London. SW1X 8QG
Telephone: 0207 235 3325
Website: www.mariecurie.org.uk

Scottish office:
21 Rutland Street
Edinburgh. EH1 2AH
Telephone: 0131 229 8332

If patients or their families wish to arrange private home care they can be advised to contact the UK Home Carers Association. This organization represents private organizations offering home care services and its members operate to a code of practice. They also publish useful guidelines to choosing home care.

United Kingdom Home Carers Association
42b Banstead Road
Carshalton Beeches
Surrey. SM5 3NW
Telephone: 0208 288 1551

Finding hospice care

If a patient wishes to enter a hospice staff should try to organize this promptly whenever possible. Some hospices will have a waiting list and patients from home may take precedence over patients in hospital as their need is often greater. Patients are unlikely to derive benefit from hospice care if they are admitted to a hospice in the last hours of life, as all too frequently happens. If a patient is nearing death it may well be kinder not to move him or her into an unfamiliar environment.

Hospice care should be used to fulfil the needs of the patient not the hospital and terminal patients should never be regarded as 'blocking' acute beds. Regrettably there is nowadays much pressure to discharge terminal patients from acute beds.

The majority of hospice in-patient care is provided by voluntary or independent hospices with some being provided in designated National Health Service units. Information may be available locally from the local healthcare trust or local telephone directory. Alternatively a good source of information on hospice services, both in the UK and abroad is the

Hospice Information Service who publish an annual Directory of Hospice and Palliative Care Services and who will provide information by telephone. Contact:

Hospice Information Service
St Christopher's Hospice
51–59 Lawrie Park Road
Sydenham
London. SE26 6DZ
Telephone: 0208 778 9252 ext: 262/263
Internet: http://www.kcl.ac.uk/kis/schools/kcsmd/palliative/top.htm

In-patient care is also provided by the following charitable organizations:

Macmillan Cancer Relief
15/19 Britten Street
London. SW3 3TZ
Telephone: 0207 351 7811

Macmillan Cancer Relief funded fifteen in-patient Macmillan Cancer Care Units in the grounds of NHS hospitals and in addition run a number of day care centres.

Marie Curie Cancer Care
Head Office
28 Belgrave Square
London. SW1X 8QG
Telephone: 0207 235 3325

Marie Curie Cancer Care run eleven hospices throughout the UK, some incorporating home care teams as well as in-patient beds.

Sue Ryder Foundation
Headquarters
Sue Ryder Home
Cavendish
Sudbury
Suffolk. CO10 8AY
Telephone: 01787 280252

Sue Ryder Foundation homes provide in-patient care for patients with a range of disabilities including cancer and in some cases also provide home care services.

Help the Hospices
34–44 Britannia Street
London. WC1X 9JG
Website: http://www.helpthehospices.org.uk/hth

An organization mainly dedicated to supporting the work of hospices. Their website includes the facility to search for a hospice in a particular area.

Useful local addresses (for personal use)

Welfare benefits for the dying patient

Anyone who is terminally ill is likely to be entitled to Attendance Allowance (if they are over 65) or Disability Living Allowance care component (if they are under 65). The patient need not know the prognosis nor do anything active about the claim; relatives or staff can take all the necessary action. The only patients who would not benefit are those getting these benefits or those who will not be discharged from hospital before death.

A claim form must be completed. These are available from the Benefits Agency. The questionnaire about the patient's disabilities does not need to be completed for people who are terminally ill unless they are also claiming DLA Mobility Component.

For social security purposes a person is terminally ill if their death within the next six months would not be unexpected and they are suffering from a progressive condition. A special form must be completed by a doctor and sent in with the claim form. The form asks for details of diagnosis, clinical findings and treatment, but not prognosis. Benefit is paid immediately. It is not taxed and does not reduce other benefits the patient might be getting. Indeed it may increase other benefits and enable a carer to claim Invalid Care Allowance.

For further information and advice contact your local Benefits Agency. Your local social work department or Citizen's Advice Bureau may also be able to help. Some local authorities or trusts also employ a welfare rights officer.

Useful contacts

The Benefits Agency provides a Publicity Hotline to keep professionals up-to-date with legislation and benefits on:

> Telephone: 0645 540 000

Advice on the benefits discussed above is available from the Benefits Enquiry Line on:

> Telephone: 0800 88 22 00

Advice about welfare rights is available from:

Welfare Rights Advisory Service
15 London Road
Kettering
Northants. NN16 OEFF
Telephone: 01536 520 387 (Mon–Fri: 10.00–12.30 hr)

Local contacts (for personal use)

2.3 Last wishes: making the most of the life that is left

Bright ideas

If you knew you were going to die in a few weeks or months, what would you want to do with your life? Would you still want to get up every morning and go to work? It is unlikely that you would choose to spend it in the often dreary surroundings of a hospital, queuing for an out-patient clinic or waiting for an ambulance to take you home.

Dying should at least give us the chance to break out of some of our everyday routines and cares. People who are dying often speak of taking one day at a time, trying to enjoy each day; to make the most of the short life that is left. Time for them is precious and we can help the terminally ill to find fulfilment in the days, weeks or months that are left to them.

Too many patients are reluctant to bother us with their worries or concerns, let alone engage us in fulfilling their hopes and dreams. We can encourage patients to express 'last wishes' and, in small ways, we can help to achieve them. Relatives, too, can be encouraged to assist the patient in fulfilling their wishes however 'silly' or unconventional they may seem.

Sometimes people express a wish to visit somewhere for the first or last time, to achieve something they have never done or see someone again who has meant a lot to them. If we want to help people to achieve their dreams we need to be imaginative and to be bold. We are often timid about asking for things for fear of refusal. Remember we are not asking for ourselves and people can at worst say no. There is a great deal of untapped generosity in the community which we can draw on. If your patient would appreciate a last visit to a football club, a meal out in a restaurant or a trip to the theatre, try asking local firms to help or appealing through your local newspaper.

I once nursed a patient who was generously supplied with a pair of binoculars by a leading manufacturer. This enabled him to enjoy his hobby of bird watching to the very end of his life. Even a bird feeder outside the ward window can provide some patients with hours of pleasure and a window to the outside world. Try having a competition for bright ideas to make your patients' lives more interesting.

At the very end of life there may be sights, sounds, smells or tastes which people want to be reminded of. The Zorzas (1980) recount how their daughter Jane wanted to smell her favourite herbs and touch a piece of velvet. Encourage relatives to provide things such as the patient's favourite music to personalize the environment.

There are a number of organizations which provide 'dreams' for dying children. I have found no similar organization for adults in this country, although some exist in the USA. Try the USA. website dedicated to 'dying well' www.abcd.caring.com

Useful organizations

Dream Foundation Dedicated to Children
Room 106
Tyne Brewery
Gallowgate
Newcastle-upon-Tyne. NE99 1RA
Telephone: 0191 222 0567

Make A Wish Foundation
Suite B
Rossmore House
26–42 Park Street
Camberley
Surrey. GU15 3PL
Telephone: 01276 24127

A registered charity which grants wishes to children with a life threatening illness aged 3–18 years old.

Starlight Foundation
11–15 Emerald Street
London. WC1N 3QL
Telephone: 0207 430 1642

Good Bears of the World (UK) Trust
Chairman Mrs Audrey Duck
256 St Margarets Road
Twickenham
Middlesex. TW1 1PE

Supplies teddy bears on request to the sick or infirm of any age. A teddy bear can be comforting to a dying person and can also be passed on to the bereaved as a point of contact with the person who has died.

Art and creative therapy

Hospices have promoted the use of arts and creative therapy in terminal care. These provide distraction from pain and distressing symptoms as well as enhancing the patient's quality of life. A number of organizations promote the provision of creative arts in hospital and hospice settings.

Creative therapies can also give patients opportunities to come to terms with their illness. In addition they can create a very personal item of remembrance for loved ones. Some hospices now also employ volunteers to help patients record their personal memoirs, either in writing or on tape.

British Society for Music Therapy
69 Avondale Avenue
East Barnet
Herts. EN4 8NB

The Council for Music in Hospitals
74 Queens Road
Hersham
Surrey. KT12 5LW
Telephone: 01932 252809

The Creative Response
The Old Coal House
Station Road
Ardleigh
Colchester. CO7 7RR

Hospice Arts
The Forbes Trust
9 Artillery Lane
London. E1 7LP
Telephone: 01732 359171

Useful publications

A publication entitled *Celebration – The Arts and Terminal Care* is available from:

Yorkshire & Humberside Arts
21 Bond Street
Dewsbury
West Yorkshire. WF13 1AX
Telephone: 01924 455555

It gives helpful guidance on 'how to get started with arts projects in a hospital/hospice setting'.

Holidays

If a terminally ill patient is able to take a holiday this can be very beneficial. There are a number of organizations which provide information and advice on arranging holidays for the sick and disabled. The Hospice Information Service provide a useful factsheet entitled *Holiday and Travel Information for Patients and Carers*, listing organizations that provide holiday accommodation.

Other useful organizations offering holiday advice to the sick and disabled are:

Holiday Care Services
2nd Floor Imperial Buildings
Victoria Road
Horley
Surrey. RH6 7PZ
Telephone: 01293 774 535

Provides information and directory of holidays for the disabled.

National Holiday Fund for Sick and Disabled Children
Suite 1
Princess House
New Road
Dagenham
Essex. RM10 9LS
Telephone: 0208 595 9624

National Retreat Association
Central Hall
256 Bermondsey Street
London. SE1 3UJ
Telephone: 0207 357 7736

Publishes information on monastic hospitality for people who feel they would benefit from a period of religious contemplation. Patients would need to still be fairly fit and well to benefit as most accommodation is of a simple standard. The service may be more appropriate to staff, patients' families or the bereaved.

Travel Freedom
Unit 2B
2 St David's Industrial Estate
Pengam. NP2 1SW
Telephone: 01443 831 000

Provides an information service on travel for the physically disabled and medically infirm.

Tripscope
The Courtyard
Evelyn Road
London. W4 5JL
Telephone: 0208 994 9294

Helpline giving travel advice for older and disabled people.

The Hospice Information Service also publish an excellent factsheet entitled *Flying Home* which gives a detailed checklist to help terminally ill patients to arrange international travel. This includes information on patient safety, insurance, special equipment and travelling with controlled drugs.

2.4 Family reconciliation and reunion

Family tracing

If a patient wishes to see a family member with whom they have lost touch, it may be possible to trace the person through a specialist agency. First of all friends and family should be involved to try to discover a contact point, or possibly an appeal in a local newspaper may be successful. It is *essential* to know the full name and date of birth of the missing person in order for a formal search to have a chance of success. Contact:

> **Family Tracing Service**
> Salvation Army
> 105/109 Judd Street
> King's Cross
> London. WC1H 9TS
> Telephone: 0207 383 2772

Some older people who served in the Second World War may be anxious to regain contact with an old wartime comrade. This may often be possible through the relevant service organization, and the Royal British Legion may be a good point of initial contact.

'Death-bed' marriages in hospital

In speaking of 'death-bed' marriages in hospital, a distinction needs to be drawn between:

(a) situations where a patient is not expected to recover or to be able to leave hospital, but is *not in immediate danger of dying*; and
(b) situations where there is an expectation or *risk of death within a short time.*

In respect of (a), it is possible for the hospital chaplain to solemnize a marriage in the hospital on the authority of a *Superintendent Registrar's Certificate* (SRC). This certificate cannot be issued until 21 days after notice has been given to the Superintendent Registrar. This procedure is therefore inappropriate for patients in category (b). Where the condition of the patient is critical and time is short, as in (b), there are two possible ways forward.

1 The marriage may take place by *Registrar General's Licence*. In this situation a civil marriage only will take place. The Registrar will attend at very short notice and will conduct the *Civil Marriage Ceremony*, which seals the marriage in law. A *Service of Blessing*, conducted by the chaplain, may take place after the civil ceremony.
2 Where those intending to be married, seek a marriage service according to the rites of the Church of England, application will have to be made for an *Archbishop's Special Licence* (ASL), where special arrangements can sometimes be made in a genuine emergency. The ASL has certain conditions which are:

(a) Both parties must genuinely desire to be married according to the rites and ceremonies of the appropriate Church.
(b) One party must be baptised.
(c) Neither party can be divorced, with a former partner still living.
(d) The parties must seek the goodwill of respective families/relatives.

The following will also be required:

(a) A letter from the doctor in attendance (not a House Officer).
(b) A letter of authorization from the Hospital Management.
(c) A letter from the chaplain which sets out the pastoral background to the situation, and supports the application. The chaplain will also contact the Incumbent, on whose parish the hospital stands, to obtain the loan of Marriage Register Books.

Where a request for 'death-bed' marriage is expressed the hospital chaplain needs to be notified at once. Even if a civil ceremony is required, the hospital chaplaincy will usually be the best people to advise on the formalities required.

2.5 Pets

Pets can be important companions, particularly to the elderly and those living alone. For some terminally ill people, the present and future welfare of their pet will be a major concern. If pets require urgent care either during the patient's illness or after their death a number of animal welfare organizations may be able to help. Some national organizations are listed below, other local organizations will be listed in your telephone directory. Some organizations have a policy of euthanasia for animals not found a home after a specified time period. This should be discussed with both the organization and the patient before any arrangements are made to hand over the pet.

Useful organizations

Animal Welfare Trust
Tylers Way
Watford Bypass
Watford
Herts. WD2 8HP
Telephone: 0208 421 8028

Has centres in Watford, Somerset and Birmingham.
The Animal Welfare Trust runs an emergency pet care scheme for the pets of elderly people during their hospital treatment and convalescence, and will also care for the pets of the terminally ill. They have a policy that no healthy animal will be put to sleep.

Cats Protection League
17 Kings Road
Horshaw
West Sussex. RH13 5PN
Telephone: 01403 261 947

Publishes a leaflet entitled *What Will Become of My Cat?* This details their scheme for arranging for a cat to be cared for when its owner falls ill or dies.

The Cinnamon Trust
Poldarves Farm
Treslowe Common
Germoe
Penzance
Cornwall. TR20 9PX
Telephone: 01736 850 291

A specialist national charity providing support for the elderly and terminally ill and their pets. It aims to keep the owner and their pet together for as long as possible and provides volunteers for dog walking and also for foster care during hospital stays. The Trust provides long-term care for pets whose owners have died. Arrangements should be made well in advance if possible. The Trust also produces a pet friendly Care Homes Register for people going into residential care who do not want to be parted from their pet.

Pet therapy

You may also wish to consider arrangements for allowing visits to a patient by their pet; this can be very therapeutic. Some organizations will also supply volunteers to provide pet therapy for patients, for example, the PAT dog scheme. Contact:

Pets As Therapy (PAT dogs)
Telephone: 01732 872 222

The Society for Companion Animal Studies
Telephone: 01877 330 996

2.6 Organizations offering practical help and support

Age Concern
Head Office
Astral House
1268 London Road
London. SW16 4ER
Telephone: 0208 679 8000

Offers practical help, advice and support to older people.

Befriending Network
6 Park Village West
London. NW1 4AE
Telephone: 0207 388 9729

Provides a befriending service to people with life threatening illnesses. Volunteers are available in London and Oxford, but the service is planned to expand nationwide.

British Red Cross

The British Red Cross provide a medical loans service for patients needing equipment in their own homes such as commodes and wheelchairs. They will be listed in your local telephone directory.

Carers National Association
20–25 Glasshouse Yard
London. EC1A 4JS
Telephone: 0207 490 8818 (Administration)
Telephone: 0207 490 8898 (Helpline)

Information and support for people who care for sick and disabled relatives and friends.

The Continence Foundation
307 Hatton Square
16 Baldwins Gardens
London. EC1N 7RJ
Telephone: 0207 404 6875
Helpline: 0207 831 9831

Provides information and advice on problems of continence.

Counsel and Care
Twyman House
16 Bonny Street
London. NW1 9PG
Telephone: 0207 485 1550
Helpline: 0845 300 7585 (10.30–16.00 hr weekdays)

Provides advice and information about provision of services for older people.
Some small grants are also available.

Association of Crossroads Care Attendant Schemes
10 Regent Place
Rugby
Warwickshire. CV21 2PN
Telephone: 01788 573 653

Crossroads is a national charity offering practical help to carers. Some Crossroads schemes offer help to people receiving palliative care. Contact the national office for guidance.

DIAL UK
Park Lodge
St Catherine's Hospital
Tickhill Road
Doncaster. DN4 8QN

DIAL UK is the national association of the DIAL network of over 100 disability information and advice services. DIAL groups give free, independent and impartial advice on all aspects of disability. They are run and staffed by people with direct experience of disability.

Disabled Living Foundation
380–384 Harrow Road
London. W9 2HU
Telephone: 0207 289 6111
Helpline: 0870 603 9177
(Mon–Fri: 10.00–16.00 hr: calls 8p per minute)

Minicom : 0870 603 9176
Website: www.dlf.org.uk

Helpline provides information and advice on all types of equipment for the disabled which can also be tried out at the centre.

SPOD
(The Association to Aid Sexual and Personal Relationships of People with a Disability)
286 Camden Road
London. N7 OBJ
Telephone: 0207 607 8851

Provides counselling and support to disabled people with sexual or relationship problems.

Useful local addresses (for personal use)

References

Faulder, C. (1985) *Whose Body Is It? The Troubling Issue of Informed Consent*. London: Virago Press.
Parkes, C.M. (1985) 'Terminal care: home, hospital or hospice' *Lancet*, i: 155–7.

Saunders, C. and Brown, M. (1995) *Living With Dying*, 3rd edn. Oxford: Oxford University Press.

Townsend, J. *et al.* (1990) 'Terminal care and patients' preferences for place of death: a prospective study', *British Medical Journal* 301: 415–17.

Zorza, R. and Zorza, V. (1980) *A Way to Die*. London: Andre Deutsch.

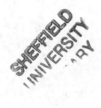

Patient comfort and control of symptoms

3.1 Introduction

Palliative care has become a medical specialty in its own right and there is now a wealth of knowledge about how to promote, comfort and relieve distress in people with progressive disease. It is beyond the scope of this book to attempt to impart that body of knowledge. What this chapter does instead is to outline a few of the basic principles of palliative care. It then guides the reader to some of the many resources in this field.

The dying patient may experience a range of distressing physical symptoms such as pain, nausea, breathlessness etc. Accurate assessment and diagnosis of these symptoms is vital. Symptoms may be caused by the patient's disease, i.e., malignancy, the side effects of treatment or by a co-existing problem such as infection. Psychological distress such as anxiety or depression can exacerbate physical symptoms. A full nursing and medical assessment is essential and this must be regularly reviewed as the patient's condition changes. Whilst drug control of symptoms is important, non-pharmacological aids to symptom control also have an important role to play. A range of effective techniques are available to treat distressing symptoms and staff should seek advice and assistance if routine treatments do not achieve speedy and effective control. The patient has the right to expect effective relief of symptoms to ensure that they die with dignity and with the minimum of suffering.

3.2 Pain

Total pain

Saunders and Baines (1995) talk of 'total pain' to describe the many facets of the experience of pain. The totality of a patient's suffering includes mental, social and spiritual components as well as physical pain. Saunders and Baines (1995) go on to caution that tackling a patient's pain demands more than the use of appropriate drugs. It is important to consider the whole person in their milieu. Emotional pain such as anxiety and grief may be related to the fact that the patient faces death. It may also be related to other life problems such as family conflict or financial difficulties. Severe physical pain can overwhelm the sufferer and make him/her feel helpless. The pain of a terminal illness can seem to be without end and without meaning (Le Shan 1983). The patient who is anxious, angry or depressed is at much greater risk of becoming overwhelmed by physical pain. Family conflict is a particularly important predictor of emotional problems in patients with life threatening illnesses (Ramsey 1992).

Pain therefore needs tackling in many different ways simultaneously. In assessing the patient in pain, it is important to assess all the background factors which may contribute to their experience of pain.

Principles of assessment and management

The Agency for Healthcare Policy and Research (1994) suggest an ABCDE of pain assessment.

A refers to *Asking* about and regularly *Assessing* the pain. Patients with chronic pain do not always look as if they are in pain. The use of pain charts on a regular basis will help to give an accurate assessment of the patient's pain (Latham 1994). There are a variety of pain charts available, the two most commonly used being verbal descriptor scales and visual analogue scales. There is an extensive literature on pain measurement and some authors favour one scale rather than another. It is, however, less important which scale is used than that pain is assessed regularly and systematically. The use of a pain chart such as that devised by Raiman (1986), which incorporates a 'gingerbread man' on which the sites of pain can be pinpointed, is particularly helpful.

Some people may be reluctant to complain of pain and fearful of analgesia. Look for limitations in activity, sleep disturbance and mood changes as additional indications of a patient's pain.

B refers to the need to *Believe* the patient. McCaffery (1983) suggests that pain is a subjective experience and therefore patients are the only authority on their pain. We need to find out from the patient the nature and intensity of the pain, when it occurs and what exacerbates and relieves it. A pain 'diary' can be helpful (Corcoran 1995; Raiman 1988).

C refers to the need to *Choose* appropriate therapies. Drugs are only part of the overall management of pain. Nursing measures to promote physical comfort are an important part of pain relief. Psychosocial problems must be addressed and most patients will benefit from suitable activities to distract them from the pain. Some patients may find complementary therapies helpful.

D refers to the need to *Deliver* therapies in a timely, logical and co-ordinated fashion. This means analgesia should be given regularly in titrated doses to make sure the pain does not return. It is important to give analgesia at regular intervals 'by the clock' and to check for breakthrough pain. There is no place for PRN medication in the control of continuous pain. It has been referred to as *'pain relief nil'* or by some as *'pain relief now and then'*.

Accurate analgesic titration can only be achieved with frequent reassessment of the patient's pain. The aim of titration is to prevent the pain from returning before the next dose of analgesia. Initially, assessment should be made when analgesia is given and halfway between doses. If slow release preparations are given, more frequent assessment will be needed. The dose of analgesia should be adjusted until continuous relief of pain is achieved. The WHO recommends a simple and effective plan for providing effective pain control (WHO 1990). They suggest an analgesic 'ladder' to tailor drug therapy to the patient's pain. This involves progressive steps from non-opioid to strong opioid analgesia dependent on the severity of pain (Fallon 1995).

E refers to the need to *Empower* patients and *Enable* them to take control of their lives. An important element of this is to set realistic goals in conjunction with the patient. It may not be possible to relieve all the patient's pain immediately. It is worthwhile finding out what troubles the patient most about their pain. For many patients a pain-free night's sleep is their first objective. Martin (1997) suggests that we need to change the culture of care for dying patients in order to involve them more fully in decisions about their care. We often pay lip service to patient participation while much of our work is still structured by routines.

Why do we fail to relieve pain?

Some patients suffer needlessly; we could control their pain but we fail to do so. Much speculation and research has occurred regarding the reasons for unrelieved pain.

Staff related reasons

- Staff may have low expectations of relief. They believe pain is inevitable.
- Staff may lack factual knowledge about analgesia (Bonica 1985). They may prescribe irrationally (Corcoran 1995). This may mean giving inappropriate analgesia, insufficient analgesic or prescribing PRN.
- Staff may fail to communicate with each other or with the patient. This can mean that staff have not shared knowledge about the effectiveness of treatment. It can also mean that the patient lacks understanding about the treatment and has unfounded fears.
- Staff may have unfounded fears that opiates will cause addiction, tolerance or respiratory depression (Bonica 1985; Tookman 1996; Twycross 1972). This means staff may delay effective treatment until the patient is *'really terminal'*. This can be a particular issue for patients with non-malignant disease.
- Staff may fail to reassess the patient's pain regularly.
- Staff may rely too heavily on analgesia to relieve pain. They fail to appreciate the role of coanalgesics in pain relief. They fail to appreciate the role of non-pharmacological methods of pain control (Corcoran 1995; Raiman 1986; Twycross 1972).

- Staff fail to give administrative priority to pain control (Agency for Healthcare Policy and Research 1994; Fagerhaugh 1974). Patients are expected to wait for the drug round. The nurse delays giving analgesia through indecision or dithering (Raiman 1986).

Patient related reasons

- The patient may believe pain is inevitable and not ask for help.
- The patient may feel they have to be stoical and put on a 'brave face'.
- The patient may be anxious about medication and believe it will cause addiction or tolerance.
- The patient may stop analgesia because of side effects.

3.3 Other distressing symptoms

Symptoms other than pain can trouble the patient. Sometimes the distress caused by these symptoms can equal or exceed the distress caused by pain. A number of surveys have taken place to identify those symptoms that trouble patients most. Finlay (1995) identifies pain, weakness, constipation, nausea and vomiting and dyspnoea as the five most common troublesome symptoms.

Such symptoms may accentuate any pain that the patient has and may limit patient activity. Accurate assessment is important, as with pain control. It is important to assess the nature and intensity of symptoms and to try to discover their underlying causes. Nausea, for example, may be caused by a tumour or a side effect of treatment. Nurses may be good at diagnosing many distressing symptoms but some are frequently missed, particularly less easily observable problems such as fatigue, insomnia, loss of concentration or depression.

The checklist of symptoms given here may act to remind staff of symptoms they may have overlooked.

Symptom checklist

Gastrointestinal symptoms

- Dry painful mouth/bleeding gums
- Nausea/vomiting
- Anorexia
- Dysphagia
- Hiccough
- Ascites
- Constipation
- Diarrhoea
- Bowel obstruction
- Tenesmus
- Fistulae

Respiratory symptoms

- Dyspnoea
- Cough
- Stridor

Cardiovascular symptoms

- Dehydration
- Oedema
- Bleeding/haemorrhage

Neurological/psychological symptoms

- Loss of concentration
- Insomnia
- Weakness/fatigue
- Convulsions
- Agitation/restlessness
- Anxiety/fear
- Depression/sadness
- Confusion

Urinary symptoms

- Frequency
- Incontinence
- Dysuria
- Bladder spasm

Skin

- Fungating tumours/chronic wounds
- Pressure sores
- Pruritus
- Disfigurement/change in appearance

3.4 Complementary therapies

Many people with life threatening illnesses may turn to complementary therapies as an adjunct to conventional medicine. Some will look to complementary therapies for cure, others for palliation of symptoms.

It is important that staff are open minded about the use of complementary therapies so that patients feel free to discuss the issue with nursing and medical staff. Patients may need advice about how to choose reputable and reliable practitioners and should be referred to the relevant organizations. Nowadays many hospice and NHS facilities offer complementary therapies as part of palliative care. Before starting a course of therapy with a private practitioner patients should be advised to check its cost and whether it is available on the NHS.

The Royal College of Nursing provide a consumer guide to complementary therapies. This is available free of charge by sending a stamped addressed envelope to the address below. Ask for *Complementary Therapies – A Consumer Checklist.*

Wendy Williams
Department of Nursing Policy and Practice
Royal College of Nursing
20 Cavendish Square
London. W1M 0AB

A useful guide to complementary therapies for patients with cancer is obtainable from Cancerlink. Ask for *Complementary Therapies and Cancer.*

Cancerlink
17 Britannia Street
London. WC1X 9JN

Many nurses have developed an interest in complementary therapies in recent years. Nurses should not try to practise complementary therapies on patients unless they are properly qualified, have the full support of managers and medical staff and the informed consent of the patient (Knape 1998).

Useful organizations

Institute for Complementary Medicine
P.O. Box 194
London. SE16 1QZ
Telephone: 0207 237 5165

Can supply the names of recognized practitioners of various complementary therapies on receipt of a stamped addressed envelope.

Centre for the Study of Complementary Medicine
51 Bedford Place
Southampton. SO1 2DG
Telephone: 02380 334752

New Approaches to Cancer
5 Larksfield
Egham
Surrey. TW20 0RB
Telephone: 01784 433610

Promotes positive self-help for cancer and gives information on complementary therapies.

Complementary Cancer Care Programme
The Royal London Homeopathic Hospital
NHS Trust
Great Ormond St
London. WC1 3HR
Telephone: 0207 837 8833

British Holistic Medical Association
Rowland Thomas House
Royal Shrewsbury Hospital South
Mytton Oak Road
Shrewsbury. SY3 8XF
Telephone: 01743 261155

The Bristol Cancer Help Centre
Grove House
Cornwallis Grove
Clifton
Bristol. BS8 4PG
Telephone: 0117 980 9505

Provides emotional, spiritual and psychological support to people with cancer and their families. Patients are encouraged to explore a range of complementary therapies.

Further reading

Rankin Box, D. (1995) *Nurses' Handbook of Complementary Therapies.* Edinburgh: Churchill Livingstone.
Trevelyan, J. (1994) *Complementary Medicine for Nurses, Midwives and Health Visitors.* London: Macmillan.

3.5 Useful resources

Who to ask for help

In cases of difficulties staff may be able to seek help from their local Macmillan nurse who provides specialist nursing services for people with cancer. Getting help for people with non-malignant disease who need palliative care can be more difficult.

In some districts a local pain clinic or hospice may be able to help or it may be the case that some staff in the anaesthetics department have expertise in pain control. Macmillan Cancer Relief may be able to advise on the services of local Macmillan nurses. If in real difficulties locating sources of advice, the Hospice Information Service may be able to help. It would be worthwhile finding out who has expertise and experience in palliative care in your locality. There are a number of information services and printed guides to symptom control but it is always helpful to talk to someone with experience in the field. You may also want to consider undertaking further training yourself, a number of specialist courses exist.

Information services

St Christopher's Hospice provide an information service for health service staff. Books and reprints on all aspects of terminal care are available by mail order. St Christopher's provide their own short guide to symptom control and also produce useful reading lists on a variety of topics. A catalogue can be obtained from the address below on request. Postage must be paid.

The Librarian
The Study Centre
St Christopher's Hospice
51–59 Lawrie Park Road
Sydenham
London. SE26 6DZ

Palliative Care Today is a journal supplied free of charge to professionals working in palliative care. Contact:

Palliative Care Today
CCT Healthcare Communications Ltd
50–52 Union Street
London. SE1 1TD

CLIP (Current Learning in Palliative Care) provide an update service in palliative care, which includes quarterly updates, a guide to symptom control and access to the CLIP website. This service is subject to an annual subscription charge. Contact:

Hochland and Hochland Ltd
174A Ashley Road
Hale
Cheshire. WA15 9SF

Membership of the *Hospice Information Service* provides an annual hospice directory, quarterly newsletter 'Hospice Bulletin' and regular updates on education and training opportunities. The Service also publishes useful factsheets and will give advice by phone. Contact:

St Christopher's Hospice
51–59 Lawrie Park Road
Sydenham
London. SE26 6DZ
Telephone: 0208 778 9252

Useful organizations

Association for Palliative Medicine of Great Britain and Ireland
11 Westwood Road
Southampton. SO17 1DL
Telephone: 02380 672 888

European Association of Palliative Care
Instituto Nazionale dei Tumori
Via Venezian 1
20133
Milano
Italy

Help the Hospices
34–44 Britannia Street
London. WC1X 9JG
Telephone: 0207 278 5668

Provide training and information.

National Council for Hospice and Specialist Palliative Care Services
Heron House
322 High Holborn
London. WC1V 7PW

Produces advisory papers and a quarterly newsletter.

The Pain Society of Great Britain and Ireland
9 Bedford Square
London. WC1B 3RA
Telephone: 0207 631 1650

RCN Palliative Nursing Forum
Royal College of Nursing
20 Cavendish Square
London. W1M 0AB
Telephone: 0207 409 3333

St Christopher's Hospice
51 Lawrie Park Road
Sydenham
London. SE26 6DZ

Provide training, organize conferences and also provide publications and an information service through the Halley Stewart Library.

Sheffield Palliative Care Studies Group
Sykes House
Little Common Lane
Abbey Lane
Sheffield. S11 9NE
Telephone: 0114 262 0174

Provides training courses, workshops, publications and audio-visual materials.

Internet resources

Association for Palliative Medicine
http://www.palliative-medicine.org/

Cancer Research Campaign
http://www.crc.org.uk

CLIP (Current Learning in Palliative Care)
http://www.clip.org.uk

Help (Palliative Care) Dundee
http://www.dundee.ac.uk/meded/help

Help the Hospices
http://www.helpthehospices.org.uk/hth/

International Hospice Institute and College
http://www.hospicecare.com

Marie Curie Cancer Care
http://www.mariecurie.org.uk

Palliative Care Watch
http://www.telusplanet.net/public/palliate/pcjourn.html

PaPaS (Special Interest Group of the Cochrane Collaboration)
http://www.jr2.ox.ac.uk/cochrane

St Christopher's Hospice
http://www.kcl.ac.uk/kis/schools/kcsmd/palliative/top.htm

Websters Death, Dying and Grief Guide
http://www.katsden.com/death/index.html.

Further reading

Agency for Healthcare Policy and Research (1994) *Management of Cancer Pain : Clinical Guidelines*, No. 9. US Rockville, MD: Department of Health and Human Services.

Doyle, D. (1997) *Oxford Textbook of Palliative Medicine*. Oxford: Oxford University Press.

Dunlop, R. (1998) *Cancer Palliative Care*. London: Springer.

Kaye, P. (1992) *A to Z of Hospice and Palliative Care*. Northampton: EPL.

National Council for Hospice and Specialist Palliative Care Services (1997) *Changing Gear – Guidelines for Managing the Last Days of Life in Adults*. Working Party on Clinical Guidelines in Palliative Care. London: National Council for Hospice and Palliative Care Services.

Penson, J. and Fisher, P. (1995) *Palliative Care for People with Cancer*. London: Edward Arnold.

Regnard, C. and Tempest, S. (1998) *A Guide to Symptom Relief in Advanced Disease*. Hale, Cheshire: Hochland and Hochland.

Saunders, C. and Sykes, N. (1993) *The Management of Terminal Malignant Disease*. London: Edward Arnold.

Tschudin, V. (1996) *Nursing the Patient with Cancer*. London: Prentice Hall.

Twycross, R. (1997) *Introducing Palliative Care*. Oxford: Radcliffe Medical Press.

Twycross, R., Wilcock, A. and Thorp, S. (1998) *Palliative Care Formulary*. Oxford: Radcliffe Medical Press.

World Health Organisation (1990) *Cancer Pain Relief and Palliative Care*. Geneva: WHO.

3.6 Good practice, quality and audit in care of the dying

Dying patients are a vulnerable group. Usually they are too ill to complain and where their relatives do complain it is usually after the patient's death and therefore too late for that patient. Quality of care for the dying must therefore be delivered first time round; there is no chance to 'get it right next time'.

Quality issues in terminal care

'Quality' is an elusive term which is usually used to refer to a degree of excellence. Opinions vary as to what constitutes excellence and staff and patients in particular may differ in their values and priorities. It is important that any assessment of quality should incorporate both professional and patients' views.

One of the most widely accepted descriptions of health care quality has been that of Maxwell (1984) who outlined six dimensions of quality: Accessibility, Equity, Relevance to Need, Social Acceptability, Efficiency and Effectiveness. These six dimensions can be examined in relation to existing research on care of the dying to give an impression of areas where improvement may be needed.

Accessibility

Accessibility refers to both physical access, i.e wheelchair access for the disabled, and to availability of services in a wider sense. Access to services for the dying is often governed by referrals from nurses, consultants or GPs. Are your patients being referred to all the services they need or are entitled to? Published research suggests that older patients and patients dying from conditions other than cancer may not receive specialist palliative care services when required (Seale 1993). In particular, 15 per cent of deaths now occur in nursing homes and residential homes and it is a matter of concern that patients referred for 'social care' at the end of their lives may not receive palliative care even though they would benefit from it. Research also suggests that care of the dying in nursing and residential homes often remains poor and that staff in these homes are reluctant to recognize that residents are dying and seek appropriate help (Challis and Bartlett 1988). Factors to consider are whether patients are referred to specialist services such as Macmillan nurses and pain clinics when appropriate and whether discharge planning is appropriate to patients' needs.

Equity

Equity refers to access to services on the basis of clinical need as opposed to other factors such as the patient's social class or where he/she lives. Have you ever examined the 'equity' of your referrals to specialist agencies? As indicated above, elderly patients and patients with non-malignant disease may represent the 'disadvantaged dying'. Some published research also indicates that hospice care is more readily available to the middle class patient (Seale 1991). Ethnic minority patients may also have difficulties accessing palliative care services.

Relevance to need

Research suggests that hospice staff are better at setting goals for their patients than staff in hospital settings and thus deliver more effective individualized care (Lunt and Neale 1987). An audit of nursing care plans might indicate areas for improvement in your clinical area.

Social acceptability

Published research suggests that patients usually prefer to die in their own homes (Parkes 1985; Townsend *et al.* 1990). Hospital care is rated lower than hospice care by patients and their families in terms of symptom control, communication and family support (Higginson 1993). It may be worth considering what steps have been taken to assess patient satisfaction with these aspects of care in your clinical area.

Efficiency

As indicated above most patients prefer to be nursed in their own homes. Effective and speedy discharge planning can lead to the more efficient use of resources and greater satisfaction for the patient and his or her family.

Effectiveness

Hospices deliver more effective control of symptoms and better psychological care of the patient (Higginson 1993; Seale and Kelly 1997). There are many areas for improvement in hospital care with regard to symptom control, communication with patients and their families, care planning, discharge planning and care of the bereaved.

Audit in care of the dying

Terminal care is a sensitive issue and this sometimes leads to a reluctance to evaluate care in this area. A first step for staff wishing to audit care of the dying might be to audit structure criteria before proceeding to look at process and outcome criteria. Guidelines to good practice can provide a useful framework to evaluate services (see Royal College of Physicians 1991).

Luthert and Robinson (1993) suggest that an audit of outcomes should include patient opinions, professional opinions and documentary evidence (i.e. care plans).

In the case of terminally ill patients' families opinions may also be important. Auditing patients' opinions is both most important and most difficult to achieve. Audit of terminal care could include the following (Higginson 1993):

1 Reviews of care plans and charts.
2 Staff meetings to review individual cases.
3 Questionnaires to staff.
4 Questionnaires or interviews with patients and their families.

Suggested standard of care for the dying patient

Structure

- The nurse involved in the patient's care should have knowledge of the following:
  - cultural and religious factors in death and dying
  - the patient's religious beliefs and wishes
  - contact phone numbers for the appropriate chaplaincy services and other religious support relevant to the patient's needs
  - legal and ethical issues surrounding death and dying
  - any specific legal/ethical issues relevant to the patient
  - hospital resuscitation policies and procedures
  - psychological reactions to death and dying
  - the patient's understanding of his/her prognosis and condition
  - the knowledge and wishes of the patient's family regarding their involvement in care (N.B. 'family' includes any significant other for the patient)
  - symptom control and the promotion of physical comfort
  - the role of the multidisciplinary team in the management of terminal disease
  - services available to support the patient and his/her family in the hospital and the community.
- The following resources should be available to the ward:
  - a range of analgesia delivery systems, i.e. syringe drivers
  - an adequate supply of supportive aids to promote patient comfort, i.e. pressure relieving devices
  - appropriate bedding and furniture to maintain the patient's comfort and dignity
  - a supply of pain charts
  - appropriate teaching aids and information leaflets.
- The nurses involved in the care of the dying should have access to the following:
  - ongoing education and support in caring for dying patients and their families
  - current literature on care of the dying and symptom control
  - specialist advice on symptom control for patients with intractable symptoms
  - support/advice in dealing with patients and their families with emotional problems.
- Facilities should be available within the hospital for relatives to stay overnight if required.

- The ward should have sufficient nursing staff to enable nurses to be able to spend time with the patient according to his/her needs.

Process

- Following an individualized assessment a plan of care is devised in conjunction with the patient and his or her family. This will include:
  - the patient's and family's spiritual needs
  - the patient's and family's social needs
  - the patient's and family's psychological needs
  - the patient's physical needs
  - the family's willingness and desire to participate in care
  - the patient's wishes regarding discharge home or to a hospice.
- The plan of care is implemented and the care given demonstrates the following:
  - promotion of comfort and control of distressing symptoms
  - prevention of avoidable problems i.e. pressure sores
  - respect for the privacy of the patient and his/her family
  - good communication and listening skills
  - relevant information giving and teaching for the patient and his/her family
  - support for the family in their involvement with the patient
  - empathy and understanding towards the patient and his/her family.
- The nurse refers the patient to other members of the multidisciplinary team when necessary.
- The nurse represents the patient's views when the patient requests this or when the patient is no longer able to voice them.
- The nurse ensures that the patient's family are fully informed about the patient's condition consistent with the patient's wishes.
- The nurse ensures that an up-to-date contact list of relatives is documented with a record of their wishes in the event of impending death.
- The nurse ensures that the resuscitation status of the patient is documented in accordance with the UKCC Standards for Record Keeping 1993.
- The nurse ensures that the care plan is updated and evaluated to meet the patient's needs.
- The nurse facilitates continuity of care on discharge/transfer and makes the appropriate referrals.
- The nurse documents all aspects of the patient's condition and care accurately.

Outcome

- A named nurse is allocated to the patient on admission.
- The patient or his/her family can state that the patient's dignity has been maintained and that the patient's physical comfort has been promoted.

- The patient's family can state that they have been supported by the nursing staff and have been given information adequate to their needs.
- The patient or his/her family can state that the patient's individual wishes have been respected.
- The nurse can state that the ward was staffed to a level that enabled him/her to give good care to the patient.
- The nurse can state that he/she had access to support and advice as required.
- The nursing notes show that the plan of care addressed the patient's physical, social, psychological and religious needs.
- The nursing notes show that the plan of care addressed the needs of the patient's family.
- The nursing notes show that the plan of care was implemented and evaluated.

References

Agency for Healthcare Policy and Research (1994) *Management of Cancer Pain, Clinical Practice Guideline No. 9*. AHCPR.

Bonica, J.J. (1985) 'Treatment of cancer pain: current status and future needs', in Fields, H.L., Dubner, R. and Cervero, R. (eds) *Proceedings of the Fourth World Congress on Pain, Vol. 9: Advances in Pain Research and Therapy*. New York: Raven Press, pp.589–616.

Challis, L. and Bartlett, H. (1988) *Old and Ill: Private Nursing Homes for Elderly People*. Institute of Gerontology, Research Paper No. 1, Age Concern.

Corcoran, R. (1995) 'The management of pain', in Penson, J. and Fisher, R. (eds) *Palliative Care for People with Cancer*. London: Edward Arnold.

Fagerhaugh, S.Y. (1974) 'Pain: an organisational-work-interactional perspective', *Nursing Outlook* 22(9): 560–6.

Fallon, M. (1995) 'Prescribing opioid analgesics', *Palliative Care Today* 4(3): 35–8.

Finlay, I. (1995) 'The management of other frequently encountered symptoms', in Penson, J. and Fisher, R. (eds) *Palliative Care for People with Cancer*. London: Edward Arnold.

Higginson, I. (1993) *Clinical Audit in Palliative Care*. Oxford: Radcliffe Medical Press.

Knape, J. (1998) 'Complementary therapies and the nurse, midwife and health visitor (The UKCC's position on complementary therapies)', *Complementary Therapies in Nursing and Midwifery* 4(2): 54–6.

Latham, J. (1994) 'Assessment and measurement of pain', *European Journal of Cancer Care* 3: 75–8.

Le Shan, L. (1983) 'The world of the patient in severe pain of long duration', in Corr, C. and Corr, D. (eds) *Hospice Care : Principles and Practice*. London: Faber and Faber.

Lunt, B. and Neale, C. (1987) 'A comparison of hospice and hospital: goals set by staff', *Palliative Medicine* 1: 136–48.

Luthert, J. and Robinson, L. (1993) *The Royal Marsden Manual of Standards of Care*. Oxford: Blackwell.

McCaffery, M. (1983) *Nursing the Patient in Pain*. London: Harper and Row.

Martin, G. (1997) 'Changing the culture of care for dying patients', *Professional Nurse* 12(7): 498–500.

Maxwell, R. (1984) 'Quality assessment in health', *British Medical Journal* i: 1470–2.

Parkes, C.M. (1985) 'Terminal care: home, hospital or hospice', *Lancet* i: 155–7.

Raiman, J. (1986) 'Pain relief – a two way process', *Nursing Times* 19 April, 24–8.

Raiman, J. (1988) *Nursing Issues and Research in Terminal Care*. Chichester: John Wiley.

Ramsey, N. (1992) 'Referral to a liaison psychiatrist from a palliative care unit', *Palliative Medicine* 6: 54–60.

Royal College of Physicians (1991) *Palliative Care: Guidelines for Good Practice and Audit Measures*. London: Royal College of Physicians.

Saunders, C. and Baines, M. (1995) *Living With Dying*. Oxford: Oxford University.

Seale, C. (1991) 'A comparison of hospice and conventional care', *Social Science and Medicine* 32: 147–52.

Seale, C. (1993) 'Demographic change and care of the dying 1969–1987', in Dickenson, D. and Johnson, M. (eds) *Death, Dying and Bereavement*, Milton Keynes: Open University Press.

Seale, C. and Kelly, M. (1997) 'A comparison of hospice and hospital care for people who die : views of the surviving spouse', *Palliative Medicine* 11(2): 93–100.

Tookman, A. (1996) 'Myths of morphine', *Palliative Care Today* 5(1): 13.

Townsend, J. *et al.* (1990) 'Terminal cancer care and patients' preference for place of death', *British Medical Journal* 301: 415–17.

Twycross, R.G. (1972) 'Principles and practice of pain relief in terminal care', *Update* 5(2): 115–21.

World Health Organisation (1990) *Cancer Pain Relief and Palliative Care*. Geneva: WHO.

Wills and end of life decisions

4.1 Wills

Patients should be encouraged to make a will. The advice of a solicitor will ensure that the will is legally valid. If a patient does not have a solicitor, in many areas the Citizen's Advice Bureau (listed in your local telephone directory) will be able to supply a list of local solicitors who are willing to visit a hospital to execute a will.

If there are difficulties obtaining a solicitor outside of office hours, it may be necessary for the patient to draw up his or her own will.

A patient making a will should be of 'sound mind' to do so and clinical staff should advise those involved in witnessing a will as to whether this is the case. Clinical staff must be mindful of the vulnerability of patients to pressure from those who may have an interest in the will. If there is any doubt as to whether the patient is of 'sound mind' or if it seems likely that the will may be contested, the patient's doctor should record his/her views on the patient's mental status in the medical notes.

If there is any dispute about a will, clinical staff as well as any witnesses may be required to appear in court. For this reason, nurses are often advised not to witness wills. You should check the policy of your employing organization before agreeing to witness a will.

Information and advice on wills

Dying without leaving a will is known as *intestacy*. If a patient is married and does not leave a will the surviving partner will normally inherit the whole estate. (The estate is all the money and property left by the deceased person.)

It is particularly important for cohabiting partners to make a will as a surviving partner may otherwise have difficulty proving a claim on the estate of the deceased patient.

If there is no surviving spouse then the children of the deceased patient will get equal shares of the estate. (However, if one of them has died then their share of the money/property will go to any children they have had.) If there is no surviving spouse or children then the estate goes to one of the following groups in the order given below:

grandchildren
father and mother
brother and sister
grandparents
uncles and aunts

In the event of there being no close surviving relatives, any other descendants of the patient's grandparents may have a claim on the estate.

In addition, anyone can make a claim on an estate if they were supported financially in any way by the person who died immediately before their death. In view of the difficulties associated with intestacy any patient making enquiries about making a will should be referred to the CAB (Citizen's Advice Bureau) or their solicitor and should be encouraged to consider making a will in the interests of their family and dependants.

Advice on wills is obtainable from your local probate registry which will be listed in the telephone directory.

A number of voluntary organizations provide information leaflets on wills, including the following.

Age Concern publish a number of relevant leaflets, including *Making Your Will* and *Instructions for My Next of Kin and Executors on My Death*. This is available from:

Head Office
Astral House
1268 London Road
London. SW16 4ER
Telephone: 0208 679 8000

Cruse publish a booklet entitled *Planning for Those you Leave Behind* about making a will, inheritance tax, funeral plans and other practical matters. It can be obtained from:

Cruse
Sheen House
Richmond
Surrey. TW9 1UR

Help the Aged provide a will information pack. Contact:

Wills and Legacies Department
Help the Aged
St James's Walk
Clerkenwell Green
London. EC1B 1JY

On the *Internet*, City 2000 On-Line Legal Information Service give advice on making a will:

http://www.city2000.com/legal/info/wills.html

Finding a will after death

If a will is handed over to nursing staff by a patient or is found amongst the patient's belongings, arrangements should exist locally for its safe keeping and toensure that it is handed to an appropriate person. Usually the will should be handed to a designated bereavement administrator or manager. A will *must not* be given to any relative by nursing staff following a death. Arrangements must be made for the will to be formally handed over to the person named in the will as executor or to the patient's solicitor.

4.2 The 'living will' or advance directive

Consent

The two key components of Consent are understanding and voluntariness (Alderson and Goody 1998). The law states that a competent adult has an absolute right to consent to or to refuse treatment however rational or irrational their decision (Dimond 1994, McHale Tingle and Peysner 1998). Anyone carrying out treatment on a mentally competent adult without their consent could face a charge of assault (Mason and McCall Smith 1999). This does not, however, give patients the right to demand treatment which clinicians do not consider to be in their best interests.

A competent adult should be able to understand the broad nature of the treatment, its purposes and any risks associated with the treatment (Montague 1996). Consent may be written or verbal depending on the nature of the procedure. With more minor procedures consent may be implied rather that explicit as when a patient rolls up his/her sleeve to have his/her blood pressure taken. In all cases treatment should have been adequately explained to the patient, it is not enough to assume that he/she understands just because he/she is co-operative (General Medical Council 1999).

The incompetent patient

A patient is incapable of giving consent to treatment if for any reason their mental capacity is affected such that they are unable to understand or communicate a decision regarding treatment. This may be through mental impairment or unconsciousness. All practicable steps must be taken to communicate the decision to the patient and ascertain his/her wishes (Lord Chancellor's Department 1999).

If the patient is unable to make a treatment decision clinical staff can carry out any treatment necessary to save life or prevent a deterioration in the patient's condition providing it is in accordance with established medical opinion (Montague 1996).

Relatives can give insight into a patient's preferences but have no legal right to consent to or refuse treatment on the patient's behalf (Hoyte 1997).

If relatives object to treatment but there is no evidence that the patient objects to treatment then the treatment can proceed in the patient's best interests. In these circumstances clinical staff would be well advised to get a second opinion as to the necessity and appropriateness of treatment and this should be documented (Montague 1996).

In situations where clinical staff feel that there are doubts about the validity of refusal of treatment because the patient has been subject to undue pressure to refuse from others, it may be necessary to apply to the courts for a declaration as to the lawfulness of treatment (Montague 1996).

Consent and children

Young people under the age of majority do not have the same legal rights as adults. Consent law for children is provided in two statutes – the Family Law Reform Act (1969) and the Children's Act (1989) (Pennells 1998). Children who have sufficient understanding and majority to appreciate the implications of treatment decisions can consent to treatment on their own behalf. However, minors do not have the same right to refuse necessary treatment and their refusal can be overturned by parental consent or by an application to the courts to treat on grounds of necessity (Montague 1996). Refusal, however, should be a very important consideration in clinical judgements about treatment and as far as possible children should be consulted and involved in treatment decisions (Pennells 1998).

The mentally ill

Mentally ill patients detained under sections 2 and 3 of the Mental Health Act 1983 may be treated without consent. However, this treatment must 'alleviate or prevent a deterioration of the mental disorder' (B.V. Croyden Health Authority 1995 cited in Montague 1996 p. 152).

In the case of *Re C*, a schizophrenic successfully applied to the courts to refuse amputation of a gangrenous foot. He said he would rather die with two feet than live with one and the court held that he understood the implications of refusal and that the condition was unrelated to his mental illness. (Mason and McCall Smith 1999).

Advance directives

Advance directives are growing in popularity in the United Kingdom following their increased use in the United States as a result of the Patient Self Determination Act. The British Medical Association have given enthusiastic support to advance directives (BMA 1995). The UKCC (1996) has also suggested that:

> Although not necessarily legally binding they can provide very useful information about the wishes of a patient or client who is now unable to make a decision and should therefore be respected.

The Law Commission suggest that there should be a *'rebuttable presumption'* that living wills are valid if they are written and signed by the maker and have been witnessed (Law Commission 1995). However, many difficulties remain in interpreting and acting upon advance directives and some of these difficulties are outlined below. This is an area where social attitudes and legal practice are rapidly changing and clinical staff would be well advised to seek legal advice when dealing with advance directives (Dunphy 1998).

Principles of advance directives

When a patient is incapable of giving consent to treatment the law assumes that clinical staff will act in the patient's best interests. The Law Commission (1995) and Lord Chancellor's Department (1997) have both taken the view that a patient's best interests includes the patient's personal autonomy and consideration should therefore be given to their past and present wishes (Mason and McCall Smith 1999).

Advance directives give people the opportunity to express their views about future treatment if mentally incapacitated at a time when they are still mentally competent. Although advance directives have received enthusiastic support from many quarters their use remains controversial.

Some doubts have been expressed about their practical value. Firstly, it has been suggested that they are very difficult to interpret in practice as they are often vaguely worded (Ersek *et al*. 1998). This is a particular problem when people use preprinted directives produced by organizations in favour of their use. It may be particularly difficult to understand the precise intentions of the patient from such a document.

Secondly, there may be difficulties in knowing whether the individual envisaged the circumstances in which the advance directive is to apply particularly if it was signed some years previously. Treatments may have changed since it was signed and so also may the patient's views (De Raeve 1993, Tonelli 1996). It is also difficult to decide whether an advance directive should overrule the patient's current feelings and wishes even if they are now mentally incapacitated. If a mentally incapacitated person expresses a wish to be treated should this be overridden by a previous advance directive?

There are further problems if a person did not leave a written directive but friends and relatives report previous conversations in which the patient expressed his/her views. Consideration must be given to the reliability of such accounts, particularly where relatives themselves hold very strong opinions about the treatment or stand to gain from the patient's death. Sometimes relatives' accounts will conflict, adding further confusion to this scenario. In these circumstances any conversations with the patient or relatives which throw light on the treatment decision should be carefully documented. In situations of uncertainty or conflict legal advice should be obtained and an application to the courts may be necessary.

Although clinical staff must start from a presumption that an advance directive is legally binding, any evidence which throws doubt on the validity of an advance directive must be considered. If refusal of treatment is likely to result in the patient's death, the advance directive should give clear indication that the patient understood that death could result from their refusal of treatment. The *Re T* case (1992) highlighted those factors which could cast doubt on the validity of an advance directive.

Capacity

Any adult patient may be deprived of the capacity to decide either by long term mental disability or by transient factors such as disturbances of consciousness, pain or medication. If the patient's mental capacity was limited by any of these factors when executing an advance directive, there may be doubts as to the directive's validity.

Persuasion

Clinical staff must also consider the possibility that refusal of treatment results not from the patient's will but from the will of others. If the patient's will has been overborne, their refusal will not represent a true decision. This is of particular importance when assessing advance directives refusing treatment on religious grounds (*Re T* 1992). In this context the relationship of the persuader to the patient is important. For example a spouse, parent or religious leader may be in a position to override the patient's wishes. The capacity of the patient must also be considered. Patients who are seriously ill are particularly vulnerable and dependent and this may affect their capacity to resist persuasion.

Informed consent and refusal

In all cases clinical staff should consider the relevance of the directive to current circumstances (De Raeve 1993). This means asking whether the patient was able to envisage the circumstances in which the directive is now to be applied. An advance directive should not be applied if it is based upon false assumptions (Ryan 1996). For example, in the *Re T* case, the patient's mother was a Jehovah's Witness who believed that there was an effective alternative to blood transfusions in her case.

There have been a few cases in which zealous religious groups or proponents of alternative therapies have misinformed the patient as to the risks of refusing orthodox medical treatment and this should be borne in mind when assessing whether the refusal is an informed one (Young and Griffith 1992). The *Re T* judgment states that the patient's right to self determination must be balanced against a public need to uphold the sanctity of life. There are a number of areas of difficulty in assessing an advance directive and the judgment suggests that clinical staff should not hesitate to apply to the courts for assistance. This has been confirmed in recent reports from the Lord Chancellor's Department (1997 and 1999).

Advising a patient who wishes to make an advance directive

In the United States there have been attempts to promote advance directives as a cost containment strategy (Scitovsky 1994) to avoid *'unnecessary'* and expensive treatment at the end of life. This alerts us to the possibility that advance directives may not always be promoted in the best interests of the patient. The Royal College of Nursing (1992) advise caution and suggest that nurses do not get involved in helping patients to draw up advance directives. It seems sensible to suggest that patients obtain independent and impartial advice from someone outside of the clinical team (McHale *et al.* 1998).

The Patients Association have published guidelines for patients wanting to draw up an advance directive. Contact:

The Patients Association
8 Guildford Street
London. WC1N 1DT
Telephone: 0207 242 3460

4.3 Resuscitation instructions

The need to initiate cardiopulmonary resuscitation (CPR) raises an ethical dilemma. Is it helpful or harmful to attempt to resuscitate this individual patient? The knowledge that the success rate of CPR is low and that in some cases the patient will die soon of their illness regardless of CPR may influence our decisions. A large British study of resuscitation found that only 39 per cent of patients survived the initial resuscitation attempt and only 17 per cent survived until hospital discharge (Tunstall-Pedoe *et al.* 1992). Survival of CPR for patients with metastatic cancer is almost nil (Bedell *et al.* 1983). Attempting to resuscitate a patient whose death is inevitable may simply replace a peaceful death with one that is painful and undignified. Birtwistle and Nielson (1998) quote the wife of a terminally ill man who was resuscitated against his wishes:

> Instead of seeing my husband's smiling face in my mind, or his sleeping, peaceful face, my only image is of what looked like a mass mugging.

In instances where resuscitation is not believed to be in the best interests of the patient a Do Not Resuscitate (DNR) order may be made. According to the British Medical Association and Royal College of Nursing, DNR orders 'may be a potent source of misunderstanding and dissent amongst doctors, nurses and others involved in the care of patients' (BMA/RCN 1993).

DNR orders are a potential source of conflict between clinical staff. Furthermore they have been the subject of public concern on the grounds that they are shrouded in secrecy and should not be decided purely by medical staff (Tomlin 1994). Research has shown that the frequency of DNR instructions varies enormously between consultants and specialties (Candy 1991). A US study of the epidemiology of DNR orders found disparities of age, race and gender which were unrelated to the severity of the patient's illness (Wenger *et al.* 1995).

In order to try to clarify the situation for clinical staff, the BMA/RCN published joint guidelines in 1993. These guidelines suggest that there are three criteria for making a decision not to resuscitate:

1 The patient's condition indicates that CPR is unlikely to be successful.
2 CPR is not in accordance with the recorded sustained wishes of a patient who is mentally competent.

  3 Successful CPR is likely to be followed by a length and quality of life which would not be acceptable to the patient.

Most controversy centres on the third criterion. The guidelines suggest that the responsibility for a DNR order ultimately rests with the consultant. The guidelines stress the need for consultation between the medical and nursing team when a decision is made. They also state that consultation with the patient is 'valuable' but they have been criticized for asserting the rights of the consultant over and above the rights of the patient (Schutz 1994). It is particularly difficult to see how the consultant has more insight than the patient into what quality of life would be acceptable to the patient. Nevertheless, the guidelines have been upheld by the courts in the case of *Re R* (1996; cited in McHale *et al.* 1998).

The UKCC have issued guidance to nursing staff regarding the documentation of resuscitation decisions (UKCC 1993). These guidelines suggest that the instructions most reflect the wishes of a legally and mentally competent patient. An area of continuing difficulty for nurses is those instances where medical staff are unwilling to record a DNR decision but where patients who are mentally competent express a sustained wish not to be resuscitated. This places the nurse in an extremely difficult position legally and ethically. It is extremely important that nurses document any discussions in which patients express their wishes regarding resuscitation as fully and accurately as possible.

The UKCC guidelines suggest that a DNR order must be entered in the patient's medical notes and signed and dated by the responsible medical practitioner. It must be located quickly and easily in the medical notes and should be communicated to all of the clinical team. A time limit for review of the decision should also be entered. Nursing staff should not enter the decision in the nursing notes until after it has been entered in the medical notes.

Regrettably there are still some instances where there is a tacit understanding that a patient will not be resuscitated but where doctors are reluctant to document this (Page 1996). This places an unfair burden on nursing staff. In the absence of an explicit recorded DNR instruction, resuscitation should be initiated if cardiac arrest occurs. Failure to do so could result in the nurse being reported to the UKCC for professional misconduct.

To conclude, it is absolutely essential that explicit DNR decisions are made and correctly documented. Nursing staff should be mindful of the need to involve patients in such vital decisions about their care and should document any conversations about resuscitation in the patient's notes.

The National Council for Hospice and Specialist Palliative Care Services publish a useful statement entitled Ethical Decision Making in Palliative Care: CPR for People Who Are Terminally Ill, which you may wish to use to supplement the BMA/RCN guidelines.

Intubation training

The intubation of the newly dead is a very controversial issue and its legal status is ambiguous (Ardagh 1997). Some hospitals have allowed junior doctors and paramedics to practise the technique of intubation on recently deceased patients, often following failed CPR. The BMA and RCN have stated that this practice can only be justified in exceptional circumstances. Their guidlines state that intubation of deceased patients:

- should almost never happen;
- can only be justified if the body has severe head, neck or facial injuries when the learner may need to practise in order to benefit future patients with such injuries;
- must be taught by a senior doctor with the relevant specialist experience;
- must only be learnt by someone experienced in normal intubation techniques;
- must not be carried out in secret (Nursing Standard 1993).

References

Alderson, P. and Goody, C. (1998) 'Theories of consent'. *British Medical Journal*, 317:1313–15.

Ardagh, M. (1997) 'May we practise endotracheal intubation on the newly dead?' *Journal of Medical Ethics* 23:289–94.

Bedell, S. *et al.* (1983) 'Survival after cardiopulmonary resuscitation in hospital', *New England Journal of Medicine* 309(10): 569–76.

Birtwistle, J. and Nielson, A. (1998) 'Do Not Resuscitate: an ethical dilemma for the decision-maker', *British Journal of Nursing* 7(9): 543–9.

British Medical Association (1995) *Advance Statements about Medical Treatment*. London: BMJ Publishing Group.

British Medical Association/Royal College of Nursing (1993) *Statement on Cardiopulmonary Resuscitation*. London: BMA/RCN.

Candy, C.E. (1991) 'Not for resuscitation: the student nurse's viewpoint', *Journal of Advanced Nursing* 16(2): 138–46.

De Raeve, L. (1993) 'Informed consent and living wills', *European Journal of Cancer Care* 2: 150–6.

Dimond, B. (1994) 'Living wills: patient choice and the Accident and Emergency nurse', *Accident and Emergency Nursing* 2: 110–13.

Dunphy, K. (1998) 'Advance directive – through a glass, darkly', *Palliative Care Today* 7(3): 24–5.

Ersek, M. *et al.* (1998) 'Multicultural considerations in the use of advance directives', *Oncology Nurses' Forum* 25: 10.

General Medical Council (1999) *'Seeking Patients' Consent: the Ethical Considerations'* London: GMC.

Hoyte, P. (1997) 'Consent may not be needed to save life', *British Medical Journal* 315:1531–32.

Law Commission (1995) *Mental Incapacity*. Law Commission, No. 231.

Lord Chancellor's Department (1997) *'Who Decides? Making decisions on behalf of mentally incapacitated adults'*. London: HMSO (CM 3808).

Lord Chancellor's Department (1999) *'Making Decisions. The Government's Proposals for making decisions on behalf of the mentally incapacitated adults*. London: HMSO (CM 4465).

Mason, J.K. and McCall Smith, R.A. (1999) *Law and Medical Ethic*. London: Butterworths.

McHale, J., Tingle, J. and Peysner, J. (1998) *Law and Nursing*. Oxford: Butterworth–Heinemann.

Montague, A. (1996) *Legal Problems in Emergency Medicine*. Oxford: Oxford University Press.

Nursing Standard (1993) 'Intubation training: an ethical practice?', *Nursing Standard* 7(44): 38–9.

Page, M. (1996) 'The nurse's role in resuscitation decisions', *Professional Nurse* 12(1): 29–32.

Pennels, C.J. (1998a) 'Consent and adults', *Professional Nurse* 13(4): 252–3.

Pennels, C.J. (1998b) 'Consent and children', *Professional Nurse* 13(5): 326–7.

Re T (1992) (Refusal of Medical Treatment) Independent Court of Appeal, 31 July 1992.

Royal College of Nursing (1992) *Living Will : Guidance for Nurses*. March, Order No. 000102, Issues in Nursing and Health. London: RCN.

Ryan, C.J. (1996) 'Betting your life: an argument against certain advance directives', *Journal of Medical Ethics* 22(2): 95–9.

Schutz, S. (1994) 'Patient involvement in resuscitation decisions', *British Journal of Nursing* 3(20): 1075–9.

Scitovsky, A. (1994) 'The high cost of dying revisited', *The Millbank Memorial Fund Quarterly* 72(4): 561–89.

Tomlin, Z. (1994) 'A matter of life and death', *Guardian* 5 October, p. 11.

Tonelli, M. (1996) 'Pulling the Plug on Living Wills', *Chest* 110(3): 816–22.

Tunstall-Pedoe, H. *et al.* (1992) 'Survey of 3765 cardiopulmonary resuscitations in British hospitals', *British Medical Journal* 304: 1347–51.

UKCC (1993) *Standards for Record-Keeping*. London: UKCC.

Wenger, N. *et al.* (1995) 'Epidemiology of DNR orders; disparity by age, diagnosis, gender, race and functional impairment', *Archives of Internal Medicine* 155(9): 2056–62.

Young, J. and Griffith, E. (1992) A critical evaluation of coercive persuasion as used in the assessment of cults, *Behavioral Sciences and the Law* 10: 89–101.

Part Two

CARE OF THE PATIENT AFTER DEATH

Caring for the patient after death

5.1 Verification of death

It is the duty of a registered medical practitioner who has attended the patient during his or her last illness to give a medical certificate stating the cause of death to the practitioner's knowledge.

The certificate requires the doctor to state the last date on which he/she saw the deceased person alive and whether he/she has seen the patient after death. The doctor is not obliged to view the body but should do so if there is any doubt about the fact of death (HMSO 1971)

In cases of expected death where there is a Do Not Resuscitate instruction recorded in the patient's medical and nursing notes there may be a local agreement that a senior nurse may verify the death, inform relatives and arrange for Last Offices and for removal of the body from the ward (RCN 1981).

Nurses *must* check the policy in their area as this varies. If a senior nurse is to verify the death of a patient this *must* be agreed in advance with medical staff.

Where nursing staff are permitted to verify the death of a patient they must record the following observations in the patient's records:

1 No heart sounds heard.
2 No pulses palpable.
3 No respirations.
4 Pupils fixed and dilated, unresponsive to light.

Nurses must also record the circumstances of the death and any subsequent nursing actions in the nursing records. The above entries must be signed using the nurse's full name.

5.2 Last Offices

The procedure of 'Last Offices' has been carried out by nurses at least since the nineteenth century (Wolf 1988). A study of nineteenth century and early twentieth century nursing texts suggests that the major principles involved in 'laying out' the patient were the control of infection and the presentation of the corpse in a manner acceptable to relatives

(Wolf 1988). The 'laying out' of the patient also allowed nurses to express the dignity of their profession and their belief in the sanctity of life. The nurse reformer Luckes (1908) cautioned nurses to remember the importance of the task:

> It is not only those about her, but the nurse herself whose nature will suffer irreparable injury if she allows herself to attend upon a death bed, or to be in the presence of the dead, either in the hospital or elsewhere, without recognising the deep solemnity of the occasion.

Last Offices is a procedure that is in part based on tradition and ritual and which has not been based on research studies. In the rushed world of modern nursing, some managers have argued that it is a task which nurses no longer need to bother with, leaving the care of the body instead to the undertaker (Speck 1992). We would do well to learn from the advice of our nursing forebears as to the symbolic significance of the Last Offices procedure. It offers a point of closure in our relationship with a patient and is the 'last thing' we can do for the patient.

In spite of the lack of a research base to the procedure, it is possible to draw up some principles of care. These are based partly on traditional practice and partly on some contingent areas of research, such as infection control and the needs and opinions of bereaved relatives.

The performance of Last Offices should take account of the following principles:

- Appropriate care of bereaved relatives.
- Appropriate support for staff.
- Appropriate support for other patients.
- Dignity and privacy for the deceased patient.
- Protection of staff, other patients and the deceased patient's relatives from infection and hazards.
- Respect for the religious and cultural beliefs of the patient and their family.
- Compliance with relevant legal requirements.
- Care and safe custody of patient's property.
- Prompt and effective communication with other wards and departments, i.e. mortuary.

These principles of care can be achieved as follows.

Appropriate care of bereaved relatives

- Relatives should be informed sensitively of the death; euphemisms should not be used (Lugton 1987), i.e. the patient has died, not 'passed away').
- Relatives should be offered the opportunity to see the body (Awooner-Renner 1991).
- Relatives should be allowed to sit with the patient for as long as they wish (Henley 1986).
- Privacy should be provided with appropriate use of screens etc.

- The patient's hand should be exposed to facilitate touching (Wright *et al.* 1988).
- A nurse should offer to remain with the relative should his/her support be required.
- The relative should be offered the facilities of the relevant chaplain or minister of religion. Religious customs should be respected.
- Relatives should be offered the opportunity to discuss the death in private with a doctor if they wish.
- Relatives should be given the opportunity to participate in Last Offices if this is requested.
- Relatives should be given time to themselves in a quiet and private area of the ward. A hot drink should be offered to them.
- The nurse should discuss the death with the relatives and give time for them to ask questions (Penson 1990).
- Nursing staff should explain all the administrative and legal procedures following the death which are relevant to the relatives (i.e. registration of death). Written information should be given to them. Relatives should be given the telephone number of someone on the ward they can contact with any further enquiries (Wright *et al.* 1988).
- Nursing staff should ensure that support will be available to relatives when they go home. A list of support organizations should be given to relatives. The patient's GP should be contacted by telephone.

Appropriate support for staff

- All professional and non-professional staff who cared for the patient should be informed of the death (Henley 1986).
- Staff who are distressed by a death should receive support from their managers and colleagues and should feel able to express their grief (Parkes 1986; Vachan 1983). Students and junior staff experiencing a death for the first time may need special support. The chaplaincy may also be able to give support to staff.
- Where staff have been particularly distressed by a death or where circumstances have been unusual or difficult it is helpful to hold a ward meeting to review the case.

Appropriate support for other patients

- Other patients should be informed sensitively of a patient's death. They should be given the opportunity to talk about the dead patient if they so wish (Henley 1986).
- Patients will be reassured by a death that is well managed and peaceful. Conversely, a distressing death can cause anxiety and depression in fellow patients (Johnston 1992).
- Patients should be consulted about whether they wish to be screened when the deceased patient is removed from the ward. They may wish to pay their last respects and to be assured of the dignified and caring removal of the patient from the ward (Wright *et al.* 1988).

Maintaining the dignity and privacy of the deceased patient

- When death occurs the bed should be screened. The body should be laid flat with one pillow supporting the head. The jaw should be supported with a pillow or sandbag to ensure that the mouth is closed. A bandage should not be used as this will leave pressure marks on the skin. The eyes should be closed if necessary by placing damp cotton wool over the eyelids. Dentures should be reinserted except in the case of Muslim patients, where this is not usually considered appropriate (Green and Green 1992; RCN 1981).
- Last Offices should be commenced within 2 hours of death. Rigor mortis may occur after this time (Pennington 1978).
- The body should be washed for hygienic and aesthetic reasons. Male patients should be shaved if appropriate. Hair should be clean and combed and arranged in the style that the patient used in life. Nails should be cleaned and trimmed if necessary. The mouth should be cleaned and dentures reinserted when appropriate.
- The application of petroleum jelly to the area around the mouth can protect against damage from stomach contents (Green and Green 1992).
- The body should be clearly identified by the use of an identiband on the wrist and ankle stating the patient's name and record number. A skin pencil *should not* be used as this is offensive to many relatives (Wright *et al.* 1988).
- The body should be straightened. In cases of kyphoscoliosis and any other cases where this is not possible straightening should *not* be forced. The mortuary staff should be informed of this circumstance.
- The body may be dressed in a shroud. However requests from relatives to dress the body in personal clothing should be respected. Relatives should be consulted about how they wish the deceased to be clothed.
- The body should be wrapped in a sheet for protection and for aesthetic reasons.
- The patient's notice of death stating name, age, hospital number, date of death and ward should be attached to the sheet.
- The feet may be secured with a bandage to ensure that the legs remain straight.
- The nursing staff should ensure that the patient's dignity is respected when he/she is transferred to the mortuary trolley and removed from the ward.

Protection of staff, patients and the deceased patient's family from infection and hazards

Prevention of leakage of body fluids

- It is essential to prevent the leakage of body fluids from the deceased patient.
- Manual pressure may be applied to the lower abdomen to empty the bladder.

- In cases of serious leakage from the vagina or bowel these orifices can be packed with cotton wool.
- If these orifices are *not* packed any leakage *must* be contained by the use of a disposable incontinence pad or nappy. Any incontinence aid used *must* be leakproof and have a waterproof backing.
- For legal reasons it may be advisable not to pack the mouth and nose in view of the rare incidence of incorrect verification of death. If leakage from the mouth or nose is expected the body *must* be enclosed in a waterproof bag.
- All wounds must be redressed with a clean *waterproof* dressing.
- Catheters, drains and cannulae are normally removed but should be left in situ if a Coroner's investigation is likely to take place. They should be covered with a waterproof dressing. Any stoma must likewise be rendered leak-proof (Green and Green 1992; Health and Safety Commission 1991).

Handling bodies suspected of being infected

- Any infection control procedures carried out before death should continue after the death of the patient. Many pathogenic organisms will continue to survive for some time after death.
- In addition, any patient who is unidentified and/or for whom there is no satisfactory medical history should be treated as a potential source of infection.
- During Last Offices all infection control procedures observed before death, such as the use of protective clothing should be adhered to. On completion of Last Offices the patient should be placed in a sealed body bag.
- The sheet, death notices etc., *must* be secured with tape in preference to pins to prevent sharp injuries to mortuary staff.
- Documentation accompanying the patient should be labelled 'Danger of Infection'. The body bag should also be labelled 'Danger of Infection'. In the interests of patient confidentiality labels must not state the specific infection involved.
- Portering staff and mortuary staff *must* be advised that special precautions are necessary before the body is removed from the ward.
- The mortuary staff may also be given specific clinical information about the patient.
- Ward staff should as far as is reasonably practicable prevent the leakage of body fluids from external orifices and wounds.
- Relatives wishing to view the body should be advised that it is potentially infectious.
- If a relative wishes to know specific clinical details they should be referred to the medical staff involved with the case.
- If there is a risk that the relative may have contracted the infection or if relatives are worried about this risk they should be referred to their own doctor and advised of the appropriate clinician that their doctor can contact for information.
- Relatives should be discouraged from kissing and touching an infected body if it is thought that this could present a risk of

transmission of infection. Handwashing facilities should be offered to relatives after they have viewed the body.

- If there is a requirement to wash the body for religious purposes relatives and representatives of religious groups must be clearly warned of the risks involved. If necessary the relevant chaplain should be contacted to discuss the matter. If the ceremony goes ahead those involved must be advised of the precautions they should take to reduce the risk of infection and they may be required to sign a disclaimer form.
- The Advisory Committee on Dangerous Pathogens (1983) have classified pathogens into groups according to their risk to workers. Precautions should be taken accordingly (see Appendix to this chapter) (Health and Safety Commission 1991).

Prevention of hazard from cardiac pacemakers

- Cardiac pacemakers must be removed before a patient is cremated because their batteries may explode causing a hazard to crematorium staff. If a patient has a pacemaker and a cremation is planned then the pacemaker must be removed. A certificate stating the absence of any pacemaker is required before a cremation can take place. The mortuary staff and bereavement office should be informed if the patient has a pacemaker and they will make arrangements for its removal in the mortuary if required. The presence of a cardiac pacemaker should be recorded on the patient's death notice.
- Written consent is required from relatives before a pacemaker is removed. If a charge is made for this procedure, relatives should be warned in advance (Green and Green 1992).

Respect for religious and cultural beliefs of patients and their families

- Different cultures and religious groups hold different beliefs about life and death. These may be manifested in different customs and practices at the time of death. It is most important that these customs and practices are respected (Irish *et al.* 1993; Sampson 1982).
- Individualized assessment of the patient is important. The patient's relatives should be consulted regarding their wishes and the wishes of the deceased patient. While guidelines as to religious customs and practices are important, it *must* be remembered that individuals will vary in their preferences and in their adherence to their chosen faith (Sullivan 1989).
- Relatives may wish to be visited by a minister of their faith and every effort should be made to arrange this.
- Religious emblems and jewellery should not be removed from the body without the consent of relatives.
- If staff are unsure of the religious requirements when dealing with a deceased patient and the family is not present then the body should be straightened, eyes closed and chin supported. Nursing staff should wear disposable gloves. Further information should then

be sought from the relatives or relevant minister before proceeding with Last Offices (Green and Green 1992).

- If relatives have a religious objection to a post mortem this should be sensitively handled. The medical staff should be invited to discuss the matter with relatives. In the case of Coroner's post mortem relatives do not have a right to refuse but may request to discuss the matter with the Coroner. A limited post mortem may be possible.

Compliance with relevant legal requirements

Coroner's cases

It is likely that a death will be referred to the Coroner in the following cases:

- Death within 24 hours of admission or surgery.
- Cause of death unknown/uncertain.
- Death is accidental or occurred in suspicious circumstances.
- Death may be the result of an industrial disease.

In these circumstances or if the nurse is in *any doubt* the following precautions *must* be observed:

- All tubes, drains and packs must be left in situ.
- Catheters and cannulae must be left in situ and spigotted.
- Existing dressings must be left in place.
- Orifices *must not* be packed (Green and Green 1992; Polson 1962).

Alleged assault/suspected homicide

If a patient dies as a result of a potentially criminal act *all forensic evidence* must be preserved. Under these circumstances the body should be covered with a sheet and should not be touched until police have been contacted.

Unidentified bodies

If the patient's identity is unknown the police and bereavement office should be informed of the circumstances of the death and will advise about the legal formalities required.

The patient with no next of kin

The bereavement office should be informed and staff should give any information necessary to assist in tracing the deceased patient's relatives.

Safe custody of patients' property

- Jewellery other than wedding rings should be removed unless it is of religious significance, relatives request that it remains on the body or removal might cause injury to the patient.

- Any loose rings or other jewellery remaining on the body should be taped in place with surgical tape.
- *All* jewellery and valuables should be listed in the valuables book and checked and signed by two nurses. Jewellery remaining on the body must be noted on the patient's death notice. Valuables include all jewellery, bank books, legal papers, will forms, money and keys. If in doubt contact the Cashier's Office for guidance.
- All patient's property and clothing should be checked by two nurses and listed in the property book. This includes any dentures or prostheses remaining on the body.
- Patients' property should be presented with dignity and therefore should be packed neatly and carefully.
- Soiled linen must be put in a separate sealed bag and labelled. Toiletries should be placed in a separate waterproof bag. Dentures, spectacles and prostheses if returned should be placed in a sealed envelope and labelled. Any letters, cards etc., should be put in a large envelope sealed and labelled.
- The property should be placed in property bags and well secured at the top. Bin liners should *never* be used or yellow bags or transparent plastic bags. *Only* property bags should be used. Nursing staff should be aware that insensitively packaged property can cause great distress to relatives (Wright *et al.* 1988).

Prompt and effective communication with other wards and departments

- The bereavement office should be notified as soon as possible after a death. They should be given all relevant information regarding the death.
- Special needs of relatives should be notified to the bereavement office prior to their attendance, e.g. disabilities, need for an interpreter.
- The mortuary staff should be given all relevant information about a deceased patient, e.g. risk of infection, religious requirements.
- Other departments providing services to the patient should be notified so that services can be rescheduled. It is particularly important to spare relatives the distress of receiving appointment cards after a patient has died.
- Other staff involved with the patient such as chaplains and social workers should be informed of the death. Do not wait until they arrive on the ward to visit the patient.

5.3 The patient with no next of kin

If a patient has no next of kin and has not left a will the first thing to be determined is who is responsible for registering the death and arranging the funeral. For a patient who dies in hospital, the health authority will be responsible for arranging the deceased patient's funeral. In practice this will mean the staff of the hospital where the patient died. If a patient dies outside hospital, the local authority is responsible for arranging the funeral. A local funeral director will be contacted to carry out a simple funeral in these cases. The deceased is often cremated. Cremation must not take place if a person has expressed an objection and any views that the patient expresses about funeral arrangements must be documented. If disposal is by burial, a common unmarked grave will be used with no memorial. The local authority or health authority may recover the cost of the funeral from the deceased's estate.

Hospitals may also register a death or arrange a funeral where a relative is unable or unwilling to do so, for example, if they are elderly or disabled. They may claim the cost of the funeral from the deceased's estate or any surviving close relative.

In cases where a seriously ill patient has no known next of kin, nursing staff should tactfully try to find out whether the patient has any surviving relatives they would wish to contact. Although it is a delicate matter, it would be useful for the patient to consider making a will. Staff may wish to broach these matters with the patient, but should be sensitive to the fact that some patients will not wish to discuss them.

Nursing staff should document details of any relatives mentioned, and in the event of the patient's death these details should be passed to the person handling the estate and arranging the funeral. Nursing staff should also try to keep records of any visitors and obtain contact phone numbers. If it is likely that they would want to attend the funeral, they should be informed of the funeral arrangements made. This includes any staff visiting the patient regularly, such as chaplains and social workers.

If it is necessary to trace surviving relatives, it is important that the full name (including maiden name if known) and date of birth of the relative is known. The Family Tracing Service can be used to trace relatives following a death.

Family Tracing Service
Salvation Army
105/109 Judd Street
Kings Cross
London. WC1H 9TS
Telephone: 0207 383 2772

If the patient leaves any money or property after debts and funeral expenses have been paid, the whole of the patient's estate will go to the Crown. Such estates are known in law by the Latin name *'bono vancantia'*. In these cases, it is particularly important to ascertain whether any relatives survive who could inherit the property. Entitled relatives are any descendants of the grandparents of the deceased patient. Reasonable efforts must be made to trace any relatives who are thought to exist. If after investigation no relatives are traced and the patient has not left a will, the estate is referred to the Treasury Solicitor's Department. In practice the department only handles estates worth over £250. If the estate is worth less than this, it can be kept by the hospital if it is not claimed by a relative in a six-year period (Treasury Solicitor's Department 1991).

For further information contact:

Treasury Solicitor's Department (BV)
28 Broadway
London. SW1H 9JS

References

Advisory Group on Dangerous Pathogens (1983) Categorisation of pathogens according to hazard and categories of containment. Cited in *Dealing with Death: Practices and Procedures* (J. Green and M. Green, 1992) London: Chapman and Hall.

Awooner-Renner, S. (1991) 'I desperately needed to see my son', *British Medical Journal* 302: 356.

Green, J. and Green, M. (1992) *Dealing with Death: Practices and Procedures*. London: Chapman and Hall.

Health and Safety Commission (1991) *Safe Working and the Prevention of Infection in the Mortuary and Postmortem Room*. Health Services Advisory Committee. London: HMSO.

Henley, A. (1986) *Good Practice in Hospital Care for Dying Patients*. London: Kings Fund Publications.

HMSO (1971) *Report of the Committee on Death Certification*. Cmnd 4810. London: HMSO.

Irish, D. *et al*. (1993) *Ethnic Variations in Dying, Death and Grief*. Washington: Taylor and Francis.

Johnston, M. (1992) 'The impact of death on fellow hospice patients', *British Journal of Medical Psychology* 65: 67–72.

Luckes, E. (1908) *General Nursing*. London: Kegan, Paul, Trench, Trubner and Co.

Lugton, J. (1987) *Communicating with Dying Patients and their Families*. London: Austen Cornish.

Parkes, C. M. (1986) 'The caregiver's griefs', *Journal of Palliative Care* 1(2): 5–7.

Pennington, E. (1978) 'Postmortem care: more than ritual', *American Journal of Nursing* May: 846–7.

Penson, J. (1990) *Bereavement – A Guide for Nurses*. London: Harper Row.

Polson, C. *et al*. (1962) *The Disposal of the Dead*. London: Constable.

RCN (1981) *Verification of Death and Performance of Last Offices*. London: RCN.

Sampson, C. (1982) *The Neglected Ethic: Religious and Cultural Factors in the Care of Patients*. Maidenhead: McGraw–Hill.

Speck, P. (1992) 'Care after death', *Nursing Times* 88(6): 20.

Sullivan, L. (1989) *Healing and Restoring: Health and Medicine in the World's Religious Traditions*. New York: Macmillan.

Treasury Solicitor's Department (1991) *Guidelines for Referring Estates to the Treasury Solicitor*. London: Treasury Solicitor's Department.

Vachon, M. (1983) Staff stress in care of the terminally ill, in Corr, C.A. and Corr, D. M. (eds) *Hospice Care: Principles and Practice*. London: Faber and Faber.

Wolf, Z. (1988) *Nurses Work: the Sacred and Profane*. Philadelphia: University of Pennsylvania Press.

Wright, A. *et al*. (1988) *Matters of Death and Life*. London: Kings Fund Publications.

Appendix: Classification of infections

The Advisory Group on Dangerous Pathogens (1983) has classified pathogens into four groups according to the levels of hazards to workers.

Group I

Organisms unlikely to cause disease in laboratory workers.

Group II

Organisms that may cause a hazard for laboratory workers but prophylaxis and treatment is available and laboratory exposure rarely produces infection, e.g. mumps, measles.

Group III

Organisms posing a serious hazard to workers coming into contact with the organism, e.g. TB, typhoid, HIV virus, hepatitis B.

Group IV

Organisms posing a serious risk of spread of infection and there is no known treatment, i.e. Lassa fever. Patients with Group IV organisms are not normally seen outside of specialist infectious diseases hospitals.

Special precautions must be taken concerning patients with Group III pathogens. Advice should be sought from the Infection Control Nurse about these patients and in any other cases where the spread of infection is thought to be a potential hazard. Special precautions are also necessary with meningococcal disease, Creutzfeld–Jacob disease and methicillin resistant staphylococcus aureus (MRSA).

Organ donation and donation of bodies

6.1 Organ donation

A national audit of deaths in intensive care in 1992 demonstrated that many suitable organs were not procured for donation (Gore *et al*. 1992). While refusal should be respected, there is concern that in many instances relatives are not approached by staff so the opportunity to donate is never offered. This is particularly true outside the intensive care setting. When organs are donated, relatives often find the decision a source of comfort (Johnson 1992; Pelletier 1992; Sque and Payne 1996). Whilst sensitivity is needed in approaching relatives, failure to approach them may deny them an important opportunity to find a sense of meaning and purpose in the death of the patient.

The usual criteria for donation of solid organs such as kidneys and the heart are that the patient is between 1 and 70 years of age, brain stem dead and maintained on a ventilator.

Brain stem death

Although there is no clear legal definition of death, it has traditionally been diagnosed by the irreversible cessation of respiration and heartbeat. However, developing technology has allowed artificial maintenance of ventilation and circulation and as a result of this and the potential for organ donation, new criteria for diagnosing death have been sought (Chaloner 1996).

Brain stem death is a diagnosis of death which has become widely accepted by the medical profession and many members of the public. There are still some cultures and religious groups who do not recognize the existence of brain stem death. This must be remembered when approaching relatives to discuss organ donation (Hardacre 1994; Lange 1992; Mayer 1997).

Brain stem death occurs when there is irreversible damage to the brain stem such that it can no longer maintain independent respiratory and cardiovascular function. It usually occurs as a result of cerebral haemorrhage, trauma or thrombosis. Brain stem death is an infrequent occurrence, accounting for only 10 per cent of deaths in intensive care (Gore *et al.* 1992; Mandefield 1993).

Brain stem death is diagnosed by two doctors, neither of whom must be connected with the transplant team. Prior to the tests reversible causes of apnoeic coma such as drug depression of the central nervous system, metabolic disorders, hypothermia or shock, must be excluded. Tests are performed on two occasions and the time of death stated on the death certificate is that of the second set of tests. The interval between the two sets of tests is at the discretion of the doctors involved (Conferences of Medical Royal Colleges 1976, Royal College of Physicians 1996).

The tests firstly elicit the function of the cranial nerves through stimulation of cortical reflex, gag reflex etc., and secondly, observe for respiratory effort following disconnection from the ventilator (Morgan 1998, Pallis 1996).

Although organ donation is associated with the intensive care environment there have been attempts to develop it as an option in the palliative care setting (Feuer 1998). Organ donation may be carried out from asystolic donors immediately after death for example; a scheme at St Christopher's Hospice involves donation after death from patients with primary brain tumours (Peters and Sutcliffe 1992). The use of asystolic donors is not widespread in this country, as the success rate for 'heart beating' donors is deemed to be higher.

Contraindications

The following factors are absolute contraindications for organ donation:

- Malignant disease other than primary brain tumour.
- Major systemic sepsis.
- High risk factors for HIV or hepatitis B or C.
- Positive hepatitis B or C surface antigen test.
- Positive HIV antibody test. (UKTCA 1993)

Donation of solid organs

Transplants are now carried out of kidneys, heart, lungs, liver and pancreas. In many cases multiple organs may be removed from a donor. In all of the above types of transplant the normal requirement is that the patient is brain stem dead and maintained on a ventilator. Age limits may vary. Kidney donors are normally aged between 1 and 70, but the upper limit for heart and lung donors is normally 50. There is no lower age limit for liver donors.

Corneal donation

The cornea is the clear transparent structure at the front of the eye through which light enters. Anything that compromises corneal clarity, e.g., disease or trauma, will interfere with the passage of light into the eye resulting in impaired vision. The last resort in treating corneal disease is replacement of the diseased portion of cornea with healthy tissue from a donor eye.

Corneal grafting is one of the most successful forms of transplantation, with over 2000 such operations being carried out in the UK each year. The demand for donor tissue is therefore constant.

There are a small number of contraindications to corneal donation. These include previous eye disease and some infective disorders. The Advisory Group on the Management of Creutzfeld–Jacob Disease (Callendar 1998) recommended that donations should not be accepted from patients with dementias or neurological disease of unknown origin.

In a small number of cases malignant disease may preclude corneal donation.

A blood sample is required from the deceased patient for HIV and hepatitis B antigen testing. Relatives must be informed that consent includes testing for these infections.

Retrieval of corneas does not disfigure the donor in any way and can be carried out successfully for up to 24 hours after death.

Donation of heart valves

Transplantation of heart valves mainly takes place in the treatment of children with congenital heart disease and can prevent early death. It is an effective form of transplantation with a high success rate. There are no problems of rejection and heart valves can be stored in liquid nitrogen for up to 10 years. Removal of heart valves normally takes place during multi-organ retrieval or post mortem examination.

Heart valves can be removed up to 72 hours after death. There are few contraindications, but the following criteria exclude heart valve donation:

- Congenital valve defect.
- High risk of or positive HIV or hepatitis B antibody status.
- Major systemic sepsis.
- Viral disease of unknown origin.

Cardiac arrest/infarction and malignancy are *not* contraindications to donation.

Consent to organ donation

The legal framework for organ donation is covered by the Human Tissue Act 1961. Section I of the Act states the following:

> if any person either in writing at any time or orally in the presence of two or more witnesses during his last illness, has expressed a request that his body or any specified part of his body be used after his death for therapeutic purposes or for the purposes of medical education or research, the person lawfully in possession of this body after his death may, unless he has reason to believe that the request was subsequently withdrawn authorise the removal from the body of any part or, as the case may be, the specified part for use in accordance with the request.

Under this section of the Act, providing the deceased has signed a donor card or expressed a wish for organ donation, a hospital can authorize the removal of organs without the consent of relatives.

In practice, the Cadaveric Organs for Transplantation Code of Practice requires the consent of relatives. This is partly to prevent distress to relatives if organs were recovered against their will. It also avoids the possibility of a legal dispute with the next of kin.

The Act also states that if the person left no instruction about their wishes in respect of organ donation this can still be carried out if *'reasonable enquiries'* show that there is no evidence that the deceased objected to organ donation during their lifetime and relatives do not object to organ donation.

In cases where patients have no next of kin, the hospital authorities can permit organ donation if their *'reasonable enquiries'* fail to establish that the deceased objected to organ donation. However, if the deceased belonged to a religious group amongst whom objection to organ donation is still common such as Orthodox Jews, Hindus, Muslims and Christian Scientists, then organ donation should not be permitted unless there is evidence that the deceased wished it. Any views expressed by the patient should be carefully documented in their notes.

In all instances where deaths have been referred to the Coroner, the Coroner must consent to organ donation (in Scotland the Procurator Fiscal).

It may be necessary for the pathologist who is going to carry out the post mortem to be present during the removal of organs. Some homicide defences have been attempted on the grounds that it was the removal of organs that caused the death rather than the defendant (Green and Green 1992).

Relatives must be informed that the patient will be tested for the hepatitis B antigen and the HIV virus prior to acceptance as a donor.

Care of relatives

Relatives of organ donors face the normal grief of bereavement. Most organ donors have died sudden and untimely deaths so that their relatives' grief will be all the more acute. Organ donors' relatives face additional stresses and strains peculiar to the organ donation process.

Research with families of organ donors suggests that families can gain a sense of meaning from the death of their relative because it has helped others to continue life (Cunningham 1993). It is important to remember, however, that in most cases this research has been done with relatives who have consented to organ donation. It points to the need to make organ donation available by broaching the subject with patients and their relatives wherever relevant. It does not mean, however, that relatives who are doubtful or reluctant to consider organ donation would gain any psychological benefit if organ donation took place.

One of the difficulties for families of organ donors is coming to terms with the concept of 'brain death' (Evans 1993). Traditional notions of death involve cessation of breathing and heartbeat and the 'brain dead' patient has all the appearance of being alive. It can therefore be difficult for the relatives to come to terms with the reality of their loss. It may help relatives to be present when tests are carried out to establish 'brain death' and particularly to observe a lack of respiratory effort when the patient is disconnected from the ventilator.

Relatives of organ donors may also suffer confusion and ambiguity about the moment of death and this can make it difficult to say goodbye. The family may be encouraged to say goodbye to their relative after the second set of tests, which is the legal time of death. Relatives may need encouragement to touch and talk to their loved one in the unfamiliar environment of an intensive care unit.

Relatives may wish to view the body after organ removal and may need reassurance that the patient will not be disfigured in any way (Johnson 1992). Some families may want the patient dressed in familiar clothes, or in the case of a child, that they are accompanied by a familiar toy during organ removal. It is important, particularly in the case of children, that families are offered the option of being involved in Last Offices. The hospital chaplain can give valuable support during this time.

After the death, the family should be given details of local bereavement support groups. The Transplant Co-ordinator will also give support and relatives should be given details of the British Organ Donor Society, who offer specific support to the families of organ donors.

Useful organizations

BODY – British Organ Donor Society
Balsham
Cambridge. CB1 6DL
Telephone: 01223 893636

Internet: www.argonet.co.uk/body

A voluntary organization to support donor and recipient families.

UKTSSA (United Kingdom Transplant Support Service Authority)
Fox Den Road
Stoke Gifford
Bristol. BS12 6RR
Telephone: 0117 975 7575

Organ Donation Campaign
Department of Health
Room 580 D
Skipton House
80 London Road
London. SE1 6LH

Provides publicity leaflets for staff and the public.

6.2 Bequeathing a body for anatomical dissection

Sometimes patients will want to *'leave their body to medical science'*. In practice, this means for dissection by medical students. Bequeathal of bodies for anatomical dissection is controlled by the Anatomy Act 1984. If a patient wishes to bequeath his or her body, they need to contact their local medical school (HMSO 1988).

Strictly speaking, you cannot own your own body once you are dead. This means that relatives have a final say in whether a body can be bequeathed for dissection just as they do with regard to organ donation.

A patient *must* express a wish during life for his/her body to be used in this way. Usually individuals complete a bequest form supplied by their local medical school. Patients should discuss their wishes with their relatives to avoid relatives overruling their bequest after their death.

In the London area patients should contact the London Anatomy Office:

> **London Anatomy Office**
> Department of Anatomy
> Charing Cross and Westminster Medical School
> London. W6 8RF
> Telephone: 0208 846 1216

For queries outside this area patients can contact Her Majesty's Inspector of Anatomy on 0207 972 4342.

It is unlikely to be possible to arrange a bequest for a patient in the last stages of a terminal illness.

The objective of anatomical dissection is the study of the normal structure of the body and for this reason anatomy departments provide a list of restrictions on bequests. These are likely to include the following reasons for refusing a bequest:

- Transmissible disease such as hepatitis, HIV or septicaemia.
- Widespread pathological disorders such as cancer or severe peripheral vascular disease.
- Severe arthritic deformities.
- Surgery involving the removal of organs or limbs.
- Post mortem examination.
- Dementias or neurological disease of unknown origin (possible risk of Creutzfeld–Jacob disease).
- Severe pressure sores or varicose ulcers.
- Artificial stomas.
- Obesity.
- Organ donation (corneal donation may be acceptable).

Some medical schools will also restrict bequests to those over a certain age limit and others will only consider bequests within a specified distance of the medical school. Following a death, a bequest may also be refused if the medical school does not have space to store the body at the time.

Procedure at the time of death

If a patient dies who has bequeathed his or her body the relevant anatomy office should be contacted. The staff at the office will contact the doctor in charge of the patient and together they will make a decision as to whether or not it is feasible to accept the bequest. If the bequest is accepted, the anatomy office will then make arrangements for transport through their own funeral directors. Following a death in hospital the body will usually be stored in the hospital mortuary until it is collected by the medical school's funeral director. If a patient dies outside hospital, relatives may find that they are liable for the cost of storage and refrigeration of the body until the bequest is accepted by the anatomy office and the body removed. In order for the body to be removed to the medical school a death certificate must be completed in the usual way.

Relatives may wish to arrange their own memorial service. The body will usually be retained by the medical school for three years.

In some cases the medical school will ask to retain tissues and organs after disposal of the body. At the end of three years the medical school will arrange a cremation service. All expenses will be borne by the medical school and next of kin will be able to attend. The London Anatomy Office holds an annual thanksgiving service for relatives and friends of people who have donated their bodies.

6.3 Donation of sperm and embryos

The Human Fertilization and Embryology Act 1990 states that informed written consent is required for the storage and use of sperm and embryos. In the Diane Blood case sperm was taken from the late Mr Blood while he was in a coma from which he did not recover. Written consent had therefore not been obtained. The Court of Appeal ruled that a person's gametes must not be stored for use in the UK without informed written consent. However, in the Diane Blood case the export of Mr Blood's sperm was allowed. If a terminally ill patient wishes to bank sperm for use after their death, written consent should be obtained stating what they would want to happen to their sperm after their death and any conditions of use (Human Fertilization and Embryology Authority 1997).

For information and advice contact:

> **Human Fertilization and Embryology Authority**
> Paxton House
> 30 Artillery Lane
> London. E1 7LS
> Telephone: 0207 377 5077
>
> Internet: www.hfea.gov.uk

References

Callendar (1998) 'Tissue donation – an option after death', *Palliative Care Today* VII(11): 4–5.

Chaloner, C. (1996) 'The final frontier', *Nursing Times* 92(33): 24–6.

Conferences of Medical Royal College and their Faculties in the United Kingdom (1976) Diagnosis of Brain Death, *Lancet* 2: 1069–70.

Cunningham, P. (1993) 'A comforting approach', *Nursing Times* 89(33): 50–2.

Evans, M. (1993) 'Moral costs', *Nursing Times*, 89(37): 34–6.

Feuer, D. (1998) 'Organ donation in palliative care', *European Journal of Palliative Care* 5(1): 21–5.

Gore, S. *et al.* (1992) 'Organ donation from intensive care units in England and Wales: two year confidential audit of deaths in intensive care', *British Medical Journal* 304: 349–55.

Green J. and Green, M. (1992) *Dealing With Death: Practices and Procedures.* London: Chapman and Hall.

Hardacre, H. (1994) 'Response of Buddhism and Shinto to the issue of brain death and organ transplant', *Cambridge Quarterly of Healthcare Ethics* 3: 585–601.

HMSO (1961) *Human Tissue Act.* London: HMSO.

HMSO (1988) *Anatomy Regulations.* London: HMSO.

Human Fertilization and Embryology Authority (1997) Sixth Annual Report. London: HFEA.

Johnson, C. (1992) 'The nurses' role in organ donation from a brainstem dead patient: management of the family', *Intensive and Critical Care Nursing* 8: 140–8.

Lange, S. (1992) 'Psychosocial, legal, ethical and cultural aspects of organ donation and transplantation', *Critical Care Nursing Clinics of North America* 4(1): 25–43.

Mandefield, H. (1993) 'Making sense of brainstem death', *Nursing Times* 89(35): 32–4.

Mayer, S.L. (1997) 'Thoughts on the Jewish perspective regarding organ transplantation', *Journal of Transplant Co-ordination* 7(2): 67–71.

Morgan, V. (1998) 'Organ donation and transplantation', *Professional Nurse* 13(4): 237–40.

Pallis, C. (1996) *The ABC of Brain Stem Death.* London: BMJ.

Pelletier, M. (1992) 'The organ donor family member's perception of stressful situations during the organ donation experience', *Journal of Advanced Nursing* 17: 90–7.

Peters, D. and Sutcliffe, N.K. (1992) 'Organ donation: the hospice perspective', *Palliative Medicine* 6: 212–16.

Royal College of Physicians (1996) *Criteria for the Diagnosis of Brain Stem Death.* London: Royal College of Physicians.

Sque, M. and Payne, S. (1996) 'Dissonant loss: the experience of donor relatives', *Social Science and Medicine* 43(9): 1359–70.

UKTCA (United Kingdom Transplant Co-ordinators Association) (1993) *Guidelines for Organ Donation.* London: Department of Health.

Part Three

CARE OF THE BEREAVED

Supporting the bereaved

7.1 The effects of bereavement

Physical effects

Bereavement can have profound physical and mental effects on individual sufferers. The bereaved may suffer a variety of physical symptoms, including breathlessness, tiredness, insomnia and loss of appetite. Existing conditions may be exacerbated by the pain of grief. The bereaved may need to be referred to their GP for reassurance and treatment.

Research has suggested that grief can have damaging effects on physical health. A high incidence of bereavement has been found amongst sufferers from diabetes, thyrotoxicosis, rheumatoid arthritis and several types of cancer (Parkes 1987/8). A number of studies have shown increased mortality rates following major bereavements (Parkes 1987/8).

The physiological mechanisms involved are not well understood but it is believed that the immune response may be depressed in the early weeks after bereavement (Bartrop *et al.* 1977; Schleifer *et al.* 1983).

Studies of the physical effects of grief highlight the need for support for the bereaved. The bereaved may also be physically exhausted by the patient's illness and the demands made on them in caring for the patient and other family members. Much informal support for the bereaved takes place within the family; this means the bereaved are helping the bereaved and those involved in the 'helper' role may have insufficient help in meeting their own needs (Littlewood 1992).

These facts highlight the need to ensure that the relatives of seriously or terminally ill patients are cared for in the hospital setting and provided with adequate support services when the patient is discharged or dies. Relatives may need reminding to take care of their own health and nutrition and nursing staff should ensure that provision for meals, hot drinks, rest and sleep etc. is made while the patient is in hospital (Penson 1990).

The provision of practical help can show the bereaved that they are still valued by those around them. Guilt and depression can sometimes lead the bereaved to neglect their own needs. Providing practical help can provide a useful role for those friends, relatives or neighbours who want to help but who have difficulty in talking to the bereaved about the death.

Psychological effects

Writers on bereavement have identified a number of typical grief reactions. These are sometimes conceptualized as phases or stages but this can be unhelpful since these reactions do not necessarily follow each other in an orderly sequence. The bereaved may experience the same emotions repeatedly at different times (Parkes 1986; Sheldon 1998).

Numbness/shock

This is often the reaction which nurses will encounter when informing relatives of a death. A sense of numbness or stunning is common in the first few days or weeks of bereavement. Relatives may comment that they 'don't really believe it has happened'. Bereaved relatives may also seem outwardly calm and detached from their surroundings. Lindemann (1944) described waves of intense distress that can overcome the bereaved during this period accompanied by feelings of breathlessness, dry mouth and a tightness in the chest and throat. It is important to realize that the shocked relative may remember little factual information at this time, although he or she may retain a vivid impression of the way in which the news was imparted.

Denial

Denial can 'soften the blow' (Cathcart 1984). It helps the bereaved person to cope for a time with the loss by only gradually absorbing a realization that it is real and final. Prolonged denial can be unhelpful and it is suggested when a person refuses to remove or rearrange the dead person's possessions or persistently refers to the dead person in the present tense. These 'clues' may indicate that the person is 'stuck' in their grief and has not fully mourned their loss. Littlewood (1992) does, however, suggest that for elderly people whose social world is very limited the tendency to preserve an ongoing relationship with the deceased is a common and realistic way of coping with bereavement. Walter (1996, 1997) suggests that the bereaved need both to let go and keep hold and that all bereaved people must develop an ongoing relationship with the deceased.

Pining

Parkes (1986) suggests that pining and searching behaviour is very common in the early weeks and months of bereavement. The bereaved may feel a sense of the dead person's presence or may feel that the dead person is nearby and be desperate to find him or her. The bereaved may experience visual and auditory hallucinations or may be troubled by dreams in which the dead person is still alive or which relive the scene of the death. They may feel a compulsion to search for the dead person. Attachment to the dead person's possessions such as an item of clothing or jewellery is also common and can give some comfort. Bereaved people may need reassurance that they are not 'going crazy' during some of these experiences.

Depression

The bereaved person will suffer a profound sense of sadness. They may find that they are subject to frequent bouts of crying and that they find it difficult to cope with everyday activities. Help and sympathy from others is important. This will usually be forthcoming in the early days and weeks of bereavement. A difficult period is often three months onwards after the death when the bereaved person will still feel an acute sense of grief but when friends and neighbours may withdraw support on the assumption that they are recovering (Lendrum and Syme 1993).

Guilt

Guilt is a common experience following a bereavement. The bereaved person may have many regrets and may feel that they did not do enough for the dead person, were not kind enough or did not succeed in preventing the death (Demi and Miles 1994).

Guilt can be particularly pervasive following sudden deaths and deaths that are not from natural causes, such as accidents and suicides. Preventable deaths can be particularly difficult to come to terms with. The bereaved may spend much time asking 'if only ...'. Although these issues may need to be explored, the bereaved may need encouragement to balance feelings of guilt and regret with an appreciation of the things that they did do for the dead person. Real guilt, as for example the person who caused death by reckless driving, may be much more difficult to expiate and the person may need special help.

Anger

Anger is a common emotion following bereavement. This can be a confusing emotion for the bereaved person, particularly if it is directed at the dead person. Worden (1991) says that anger comes from a sense of frustration that the death could not be prevented and cannot be mitigated.

Anger can also lead the individual to blame medical and nursing staff for failing to treat the illness or for causing unnecessary suffering to the deceased. It is important, however, to listen carefully to bereaved people who address this anger to staff. The bereaved may have legitimate reasons for complaint. Many of the cases referred to the Health Service Commissioner are made by bereaved relatives and a substantial proportion are upheld as genuine. A satisfactory resolution of such a complaint is important for all concerned and will assist the bereaved in coming to terms with their grief.

When there is no specific focus for anger it may lead to a general demeanour of hostility and resentment towards others. This can be an impediment to the individual receiving help and is often difficult to overcome.

A danger arises when the individual directs anger inwards. This can lead to self-harm, self-neglect or suicide, and intervention may be necessary.

Anxiety

Anxiety and panic attacks are common following bereavement. This may focus on a fear that the bereaved person will be unable to cope with the loss or a fear of their own death. Sometimes anxiety is diffuse and seems to have no focus. Some bereaved people may develop phobias. Prolonged and uncontrollable anxiety suggest that the bereaved individual needs professional help.

The practical effects

Bereaved people may need much practical assistance. In the early days they may require help in dealing with administrative and legal formalities and funeral arrangements.

The bereaved often suffer financial problems as well as a loss of practical and social support. Widows and widowers with children may have special problems with child care. The bereaved may also have difficulties in dealing with new social activities and obligations.

7.2 The 'tasks of mourning'

Worden (1991) suggests that bereavement can usefully be conceptualized as four 'tasks' which have to be completed if the individual is to come to terms with their loss. Conceptualizing these as 'tasks' suggests ways in which the health professional or counsellor can facilitate the mourning process.

Task I: To accept the reality of the loss

The bereaved person has to come face to face with the reality that the person is dead, is gone and will not return. The bereaved must accept that reunion is impossible, at least in this life. The actions of health professionals immediately after a death can help the bereaved to accept this reality. It is important to use plain language: the patient has died not 'passed away'. The relatives should be encouraged (but not forced) to view the body. Time spent talking about the death now can help the bereaved later on. The staff should answer questions fully and encourage relatives to ask questions and discuss the death. It is helpful for relatives to have a point of contact in the hospital to come back to subsequently with any unanswered questions or worries about the death. Relatives often need to 'relive' the events of the death over and over again in order to come to terms with its reality and small details can assume a great importance in this process.

Subsequently the bereaved will need time to talk about the events surrounding the death and if they lack social contact and support they may need the support of a bereavement counsellor or bereavement group to do this.

Task II: To work through the pain of grief

Parkes (1986) states that 'if it is necessary for the bereaved person to go through the pain of grief in order to get grief work done then anything that continually allows the person to avoid or suppress the pain can be expected to prolong the course of mourning'.

People may try to avoid experiencing the pain of grief by cutting off their feelings and avoiding painful thoughts. Worden (1991) suggests that the bereaved must be helped to identify and ventilate their feelings. Apart from pain these may include anger, guilt, helplessness and frustration. Encouraging the bereaved to talk about the death can help them to work through these feelings.

Penson (1990), however, warns that nurses must think carefully before encouraging relatives to express their grief, particularly in the hospital setting. If we actively solicit expressions of grief we must be prepared to carry it through and know that we have the time and skills to support the bereaved. We must not offer what we cannot or will not give. This does not mean that we should not show our concern but there will be times when it is more appropriate for nurses to refer relatives to others for counselling and support.

Task III: To adjust to an environment in which the deceased is missing

The bereaved must adjust to the fact that their world is now changed. The roles that the deceased played are now missing. The bereaved person must learn to adjust to this new situation, fulfil new roles and readjust his/her outlook on life. The bereaved may need help to explore life without the deceased and make decisions about the future. They should, however, be discouraged from making any major decisions such as moving house too soon after the death.

Task IV: To emotionally relocate the deceased and move on with life

The bereaved do not have to give up their relationship with the deceased but need to find an appropriate place for the dead person in their lives that allows them to go on living in the world. This may mean making new relationships or simply engaging in new activities and interests.

The bereaved may need encouragement to take up new occupations without seeing them as a betrayal of the deceased. This can be difficult to achieve, especially for the older person whose opportunities for new activities may be very restricted. Continuing support is needed to enable the bereaved to make this adjustment.

Nursing staff are likely to come into contact with the bereaved often in their professional lives. They can try to use their contact with the bereaved to help them to come to terms with their loss. Thoughtful care of the bereaved immediately after a death can help in achieving Task I. Nursing staff need to be aware of those factors which can lead to complicated grief and prolonged mourning and should refer relatives for appropriate help and support.

7.3 Risk factors in bereavement

A number of factors have been associated with a poor outcome after bereavement. In cases where nurses feel that the relatives may be at risk, efforts must be made to arrange ongoing professional help for the bereaved.

Risk factors associated with the circumstances of the death

Unexpected death can cause a particular risk of prolonged mourning. The bereaved may have special difficulties in accepting the reality of the loss. Deaths from accidents, suicide or homicide are especially difficult to come to terms with. Death may also be unexpected where the patient had a long illness but the bereaved person was not aware of the diagnosis or prognosis.

Deaths that might have been avoided or are unexplained also cause particular difficulties, as, for example, cot deaths.

Risk factors associated with the bereaved person

Individuals who have had other recent losses may find another bereavement especially hard to deal with, as may people who have found it hard to come to terms with bereavement in the past. A previous history of stress related illness or mental health problems may also mean that the bereaved person is at risk. Physical ill health may also make it hard to cope with bereavement.

Bereavement may be especially difficult for young children and adolescents. People with learning disabilities and the elderly confused have special difficulties in coming to understand and accept a loss, which are often overlooked.

Risk factors associated with the bereaved person's relationship with the deceased

Bereaved people who have had an ambivalent relationship with the deceased may have difficulty coming to terms with the loss. For example, individuals whose relatives have died from Alzheimer's disease may have very mixed feelings about the death, which they find hard to resolve.

Relationships that have been characterized by conflict can lead to complicated grief, as can relationships where one partner was very dependent on the other.

Risk factors associated with the bereaved person's environment

Bereaved people who report that they have little social support can be particularly at risk (Parkes 1987/8). This includes both the socially isolated person and the person who has family and friends but finds them unhelpful. Maddison *et al.* (1967) found that a strong predictor of poor outcome was the bereaved person's perception that his or her family were lacking in understanding. Littlewood (1992) reports that bereavement can often lead to family conflict.

Grief may also be difficult to mourn if it is unspeakable (Worden 1991). This can happen when the death is stigmatized, as in the case of suicides, or where the bereaved person's relationship with the deceased was hidden, as in some homosexual relationships (Maxwell 1996).

Other social stresses such as poverty and financial and practical difficulties can also give rise to complicated grief reactions.

7.4 Resources about bereavement

The following organizations provide helpful leaflets on bereavement.

Cruse has a variety of leaflets for the bereaved and those who care for them. These are available free or at a small cost. Publication list from:

> **Cruse Bereavement Care**
> Cruse House
> 126 Sheen Road
> Richmond
> Surrey. TW9 1VR
> Telephone: 0208 940 4818

The *Royal College of Psychiatrists* have produced a useful short leaflet for the general public on bereavement. This is available free from:

> **Help is at Hand Leaflets**
> PO Box 19
> Basingstoke
> Hants RG26 5BR

MIND have produced a helpful leaflet entitled *Understanding Bereavement*. This is available from:

> **MIND Mail Order Service**
> 15–19 Broadway
> Stratford
> London. E15 4BQ
> Telephone: 0208 519 2122 Ext: 223

Bereavement literature

There are a number of books, novels and autobiographies which contain advice, information or personal accounts of grief, which bereaved people have found helpful. A selection of these books is listed below.

*Age Concern and Cruse (1986) *Survival Guide for Widows*. Darton Longman and Todd.

*Collick, Elizabeth (1986) *Through Grief: The Bereavement Journey.* Darton Longman and Todd/Cruse.
Hill, Susan (1977) *In the Springtime of the Year.* Penguin.
Hora, Sandra (1989) *Coping with Bereavement.* Thorsons Publishers.
*Jones, Mary (1988) *Secret Flowers.* Womens Press.
Lake, Tony (1984) *Living with Grief.* Sheldon Press.
*Lewis, C.S. (1961) *A Grief Observed.* Faber & Faber.
Lively, Penelope (1985) *Perfect Happiness.* Penguin.
Monaghan, L. (1998) *Time to Say Goodbye.* Lutterworth Press.
Taylor, Liz Macneil (1983) *Living with Loss.* Fontana.
Trobisch, Ingrid (1985) *Learning to Walk Alone.* Intervarsity Press.
Truman, Jill (1988) *Letter to My Husband.* Hodder & Stoughton.
*Whittaker, Agnes (1984) *All In the End Is Harvest: an Anthology for Those Who Grieve.* Darton Longman & Todd.
Wylie, Betty Jane (1986) *Beginnings: A Book for Widows.* Unwin Paperbacks.

*Available from Cruse.

7.5 Helping bereaved children

Children have special needs when they are bereaved. Children feel grief in the same way as adults but their understanding of death depends on their level of cognitive development (Worden 1991). Children may have difficulties in expressing their unhappiness and may feel guilty about upsetting other surviving members of their family if they do so. Adult members of the family may have their own grief to deal with and the child may have a special need for someone outside the family with whom they can discuss their feelings. Very young children may express their feelings nonverbally or through play. It is important that young children are involved and not excluded when someone is dying; it should not be assumed that they do not know what is going on. Decisions about issues such as viewing the body or attending the funeral should be made on the basis of the child's needs and wishes rather than abstract rules about what 'ought' to be done.

Resources

There are a number of useful resources for professionals dealing with bereaved children.

The *National Society for Promoting Religious Education* publish an excellent booklet for teachers on the bereaved child: *The Bereaved Child: A Guide for Teachers and Leaders* (by Wendy Duffy) which provides sensitive, useful and practical guidance for anyone dealing with bereaved children. Available from:

The National Society
Church House
Great Smith Street
LONDON. SW1 3NZ
Telephone: 0207 222 1672

The social work department of St Christopher's Hospice produce two sensitively written and illustrated booklets for bereaved children. These are entitled *Someone Special Has Died* and *Your Parent has Died*. They also provide a thoughtfully designed scrap book for children to complete about someone close to them who is ill. This is entitled *My Book About ...* These resources are available from:

The Study Centre
St Christopher's Hospice
51–59 Lawrie Park Road
Sydenham
London. SE26 6DZ

Cruse provide a booklet for parents entitled *When Children Grieve* and two booklets for older children entitled *My Father Died* and *My Mother Died.* Contact:

Cruse Bereavement Care
Cruse House
126 Sheen Road
Richmond
Surrey TW9 1VR

Cancerlink have produced a useful booklet entitled *Talking to Children when an Adult has Cancer.* Available from:

Cancerlink
17 Britannia Street
London WC1X 9JN

Books for bereaved children

A number of books have been produced for children dealing with death and bereavement. These may be helpful, particularly if they are read with the child. A selection of these books is available from most public libraries, many of whom keep a small special collection of books on this subject.

Books for younger children
Althea (1982) *When Uncle Bob Died* [Picture book]. Dinosaur Publications.
Burningham, John (1984) *Granpa* [Picture book]. Cape.
Stickney, Doris (1984) *Waterbugs and Dragonflies: Explaining Death to Children.* Mowbray.
Varley, Susan (1985) *Badger's Parting Gifts.* Picture Lions.
Viorst, Judith (1971) *The Tenth Good Thing about Barney.* Collins.
White, R. (1952) *Charlotte's Web.* Puffin.

Older children
Bowler, Tim (1997) *River Boy*. Oxford University Press.
Little, J. (1985) *Mama's Going to Buy You a Mocking Bird*. Puffin.
Lowry, Lois (1990) *A Summer to Die*. Lions.
Marino, Jan (1989) *Eighty Steps to September*. Blackie.
Paterson, K. (1982) *Bridge to Terebithia*. Gollancz.

Further reading about child bereavement

Bending, M. (1993) *Caring for Bereaved Children*. Richmond, Surrey: Cruse
(available from Cruse).
Couldrick, A. (1990) *Grief and Bereavement*. Oxford: Sobell Publications.
Couldrick, A. (1991) *When Your Mum or Dad Has Cancer*. Oxford: Sobell
Publications.
The latter two are available from:

> **Sir Michael Sobell House**
> Macmillan Continuing Care Unit
> Churchill Hospital
> Headington
> Oxford. OX3 7LJ

Jewett, C. (1984) *Helping Children Cope With Separation and Loss*. Batsford
(available from St Christopher's Study Centre as detailed above).
Krementz, J. (1981) *How It Feels When a Parent Dies*. Gollancz (available
from Cruse or St Christopher's Study Centre).
Wells, R. (1988) *Helping Children Cope With Grief*. Sheldon Press.

Helpful organizations

> **Childline**
> FREEPOST 1111
> London. N1 0B7
> Telephone: 0800 11 11
>
> 24 hour telephone counselling service for children in trouble.
>
> **The Family Welfare Association**
> 501–505 Kingsland Road
> Dalston
> London. E8 4AN
> Telephone: 0207 254 6251
>
> **NCH Careline**
> c/o National Childrens Home
> Ilford High Road
> Ilford
> Essex. 1G1 1QP
>
> Provides help for children and families in trouble.

National Council for One Parent Families
255 Kentish Town Road
London. NW5 2LX
Telephone: 0207 267 1361

7.6 Support organizations for the bereaved

Accident Legal Advice Service
Freepost
London. WC2A 1BR
Telephone: 0171 242 2430

Participating solicitors will offer a free consultation to establish whether a client has a case for claiming compensation.

Action for Victims of Medical Accidents
Bank Chambers
1 London Road
Forest Hill
London. SE23 3TP
Telephone: 0208 291 2793

Gives legal advice on cases of medical negligence and error.

Age Concern
Head Office
Astral House
1268 London Road
London. SW16 4EB
Telephone: 0208 679 8000

Gives help to anyone over 60. In some areas Age Concern run bereavement counselling services.

Campaign Against Drinking and Driving (CADD)
c/o Mrs Marie Cape
85 Jesmond Road
Newcastle upon Tyne. NE2 1NH

Offers support to families who have suffered a death as a result of drunken driving.

Child Death Helpline
Bereavement Services Department
Great Ormond Street Hospital for Children
NHS Trust
London. WC1N 3JH
Telephone: 0207 813 8551 (Office)
Helpline: 0800 282 986 (19.00–22.00 hr)

Child Bereavement Trust
Harleyford Estate
Henley Road
Marlow. SL7 2DX
Telephone: 01628 488 101

Provides help for bereaved families and training for health professionals.

Church Army Counselling Service

A non-denominational service offering individual counselling in London, Manchester and Sheffield.

London:
10 Daventry Street
London. NW15 NX
Telephone: 0207 723 0573

Manchester:
Central Hall
Oldham Street
Manchester. M1 1JT
Telephone: 0161 236 1081

Sheffield:
30 Montrose Road
Sheffield. S7 2EE
Telephone: 01742 585 360

Cruse – Bereavement Care
Cruse House
126 Sheen Road
Richmond
Surrey. TW9 1UR
Telephone: 0208 940 4818
Helpline: 0208 332 7227

A nationwide service of bereavement counselling, advice, publications and training.

Compassionate Friends
53 North Street
Bristol. BS3 1EN
Telephone: 0117 966 5202

Offers support nationwide to bereaved parents.

The Foundation for the Study of Infant Deaths
14 Halkin Street
London. SW1X 7DP
Telephone: 0207 235 0965 (Office)
Helpline: 0207 235 1721 (24 hours)

Support and information for bereaved parents and fundraising for research into cot deaths.

Help the Aged
St James Walk
London. EC1
Seniorline: 0800 650065 (09.00–16.00 hr Mon–Fri)

Telephone Hotline for the elderly.

Inquest
Alexandra National House
330 Seven Sisters Road
Finsbury Park
London. N4 2PJ
Telephone: 0208 802 7430

Support for the bereaved when a death results in a Coroner's inquest.

Jewish Bereavement Counselling Service
PO Box 6748
London. N3 3BX
Telephone: 0208 349 0839

Lesbian and Gay Bereavement Project
Vaughan M Williams Centre
Colindale Hospital
London. NW9 5HG
Telephone: 0208 455 8894

Offers support and advice to the bereaved partners of gays and lesbians.

Miscarriage Association
c/o Clayton Hospital
Northgate
Wakefield
West Yorkshire. WF1 3JS

National Association of Widows
54–57 Allison Street
Digbeth
Birmingham. B5 5TH
Telephone: 0121 643 8348

Offers friendship, support and advice to widows and their families.

National Association of Bereavement Services
20 Norton Folgate
London. E1 6DB
Telephone: 0207 247 0617 (Administration)
Telephone: 0207 247 1080 (Referrals)

Publishes a directory of bereavement services throughout the UK.

Relate (formerly the Marriage Guidance Council)
National Office
Herbert Gray College
Little Church Street
Rugby. CU21 3AP
Telephone: 01788 73241

Offers confidential counselling on all aspects of relationships including bereavement.

SSAFA Forces Help
19 Queen Elizabeth Street
London. SE1 2LP
Telephone: 0207 403 8783

Gives advice to ex-servicemen and women and their dependants.

Samaritans
10 The Grove
Slough. SL1 1QP
Telephone: 01753 532713
Helpline: 0345 90 90 90 (24 hours)

Confidential help for anyone with troubles in their life.

The Stillbirth and Neonatal Death Society (Sands)
28 Portland Place
London. W1N 4DE
Telephone: 0207 436 7940 (General Enquiries)
Helpline: 0207 436 5881

Support After Murder and Manslaughter (SAMM)
Cranmer House
39 Brixton Road
London. SW9 6DZ
Telephone: 0207 735 3838

An organization offering support, sympathy and advice to the family and friends of victims of murder and manslaughter.

Survivors of Bereavement by Suicide (SOBS)
82 Arcon Drive
Anlaby Road
Hull. HU4 6AD
Telephone: 01482 565 387

Victim Support
(National Office)
Cranmer House
39 Brixton Road
London. SW9 6DZ
Telephone: 0207 587 1162 (Referrals)
Telephone: 0207 735 9166 (General Enquiries)

Victim Support Scotland:
14 Frederick Street
Edinburgh
EH2 2HB
Telephone: 0131 225 7779

Victim Support Northern Ireland:
Annsgate House
70/74 Ann Street
Belfast. BT1 4EH
Telephone: 028 902 44039

Victim Supportline:
PO Box 11431
London. SW9 6ZH
Telephone: 0845 30 30 900 (09.00–21.00 hr)

Victim support offers help to victims of crime and their families. It also provides information and training including a useful booklet for health professionals entitled *Treating Victims of Crime.*

War Widows Association of Great Britain
17 The Earl's Court
Coventry
CV3 5ES
Telephone: 02476 503 298

Gives advice to war widows and their dependants.

Local organizations (for personal use)

7.7 Good practice, quality and audit in care of the bereaved

There is very little published research or audit activity indicating whether care of the bereaved is of an acceptable standard. What information does exist indicates some possible problems with existing services. Following Maxwell's (1984) six dimensions of quality, we can identify some potential problems.

Accessibility and equity

Access to follow up support for the bereaved is variable. Much bereavement counselling is provided on a voluntary basis by organizations such as Cruse or by health professionals in addition to their normal duties. Referral to these services is patchy as is their provision in different localities, since they depend largely on individual good will and commitment (Wright *et al.* 1988).

Practising members of specific faiths may derive comfort from the support of hospital chaplains but this is not available to everyone. Members of ethnic minorities have specific needs which are often not met by existing services. Hospices and palliative care services generally have more effective arrangements for follow up support (Faulkner 1993).

Wright *et al.* (1988) suggest that all relatives are offered an opportunity to return to the hospital to discuss the death and are given a contact phone number. Schemes providing follow up contact with relatives to find out how they are coping have been initiated successfully by Accident and Emergency departments (McGuinness 1986) and hospices (Wright *et al.* 1988). All relatives should be given written information that includes a contact number and the addresses of support organizations.

Follow up services from the primary health care team are dependent on prompt communication from hospital staff. Often this is lacking and relatives are devoid of professional support when they are most distressed. This distress can be compounded if services to the deceased patient have not been cancelled by hospital staff. Prompt communication with the GP and all other agencies involved is essential for effective bereavement care.

Relevance to need

Bereavement brings the risk of deterioration in health status. Most people will eventually recover from their grief but some will experience long term psychological or physical health problems. It is important to identify those most at risk. The most accurate predictor of those at risk is a lack of perceived social support (Raphael 1977). Many hospices use follow up contacts or questionnaires which identify those in need of help but this is a service which most acute services have yet to develop.

Social acceptability

A common complaint from bereaved relatives is poor communication. Many bereaved relatives have also reported unsympathetic attitudes on the part of hospital staff (Wright *et al.* 1988). Regrettably one research study reported that bereaved relatives found the police more sympathetic than doctors or nurses (Finlay and Dallimore 1991). Many relatives also reported that interviews with staff were rushed and that they received little comfort or support.

Efficiency and effectiveness

The most important area where efficiency and effectiveness can be improved is in improved communication both between staff and with bereaved relatives.

Some mechanism for follow up support would improve the effectiveness of care of bereaved relatives and reduce subsequent morbidity.

A suggested standard of care for supporting the bereaved

Throughout, 'relative' refers to any significant other for the patient.

Structure

- The nurses involved in the care of the patient and his/her family will have knowledge of the following:
  - the social and psychological effects of bereavement, normal and abnormal grief reactions
  - the support systems available to the bereaved within the hospital and the community
  - the family's religious and cultural beliefs concerning death and dying
  - the role of the multidisciplinary team in the management of bereavement
  - practical and legal issues following death, i.e. wills, death certification etc.
- The nurses involved with bereaved relatives will have developed appropriate communication and listening skills.
- The nurses involved with bereaved relatives will have access to the bereavement administrator for practical advice on the administrative issues surrounding a death.
- The nurses involved with bereaved relatives will have access to continuing education and support regarding loss and bereavement.
- The chaplaincy service will be available for spiritual support.
- Members of the multidisciplinary team will be available for information and support where appropriate.
- The nurse will have access to up-to-date written information and research on bereavement and bereavement support groups.
- A quiet room will be available which ensures privacy for the relatives.
- Tea/coffee-making facilities will be available on the ward.
- The ward will be staffed to a level which allows staff to take time out to spend with bereaved relatives.

Process

- Nurses keep an accurate and up-to-date record of relatives' and patients' wishes about what should be done and who should be called at the time of death or when death is imminent.

- Relatives are called to the hospital or informed of a death in a sensitive manner. Relatives are informed of an expected death by phone only when there is prior agreement that this will occur.
- Relatives are greeted on arrival on the ward by a member of the nursing staff.
- Where an interpreter/linkworker is needed every effort is made to arrange this prior to the relatives' arrival on the ward.
- The qualified nurse spends time with the relatives and answers their questions accurately and sensitively.
- Relatives are offered an opportunity to talk to an appropriate doctor about the circumstances surrounding the death.
- Relatives are offered refreshments by a member of staff.
- Relatives are given the opportunity to spend time alone in a private room if required.
- The nurse encourages relatives to remain for as long as they require with a patient who has just died. A nurse offers to accompany them if they wish.
- The qualified nurse informs the relatives about the administrative procedures following death. Accurate verbal and written information is given to relatives.
- The qualified nurse informs the relatives of relevant support services which they can contact. If necessary the nurse liaises with the appropriate agencies.
- The qualified nurse discusses the patient's and relatives' religious requirements and contacts the relevant chaplain or religious representative if required.
- The qualified nurse checks the support available to the relative on leaving hospital. If the relative is returning to an empty home the nurse offers to contact an appropriate person to accompany them.
- The qualified nurse gives the relatives a contact phone number in case of any further queries following the death.

Outcome

- The relatives state that they were treated in a sensitive and caring manner and given adequate support.
- The relatives state that the handling of the death by nursing staff did not cause them any additional distress.
- The relatives state that they were given opportunities for privacy and offered refreshments.
- The relatives state that they were able to spend as much time as they wished with the deceased.
- The relatives state that they were given correct information regarding procedures following the death.
- The bereavement administrator/registrar confirms that the relatives attended his office at an appropriate time and with the correct information.
- The nurse confirms that she was able to spend time with the relatives and provide support and information.

- The nurse confirms that she was able to obtain an interpreter/link-worker when required.
- The nurse confirms that she was able to contact an appropriate chaplain when required.
- The nurse confirms that a private area of the ward was available when required and that tea/coffee-making facilities were available.

References

Bartrop, R.W. *et al.* (1977) 'Depressed lymphocyte function after bereavement', *Lancet* i: 834–6.

Brady, T. (1999) 'When someone close dies', *Palliative Care Today* 7(4): 40–1.

Cathcart, F. (1984) 'Bereavement', in Doyle, D. (ed.) *Palliative Care: The Management of Far Advanced Illness.* London: Croom Helm.

Demi, A.S. and Miles, M.S. (1994) 'Bereavement guilt', in Corless, I. *et al.* (eds) *Dying, Death and Bereavement. Theoretical Perspectives and Other Ways of Knowing.* Boston: Jones and Bartlett.

Faulkner, A. (1993) 'Developments in bereavement services', in Clark, D. (ed.) *The Future of Palliative Care.* Milton Keynes: Open University Press.

Finlay, I. and Dallimore, D. (1991) 'Your child is dead', *British Medical Journal* i: 1470–2.

Jones, A. (1989) 'Bereavement counselling, applying ten principles', *Geriatric Medicine* September: 55–8.

Lendrum, S. and Syme, G. (1993) *Gift of Tears.* London: Routledge.

Lindemann, E. (1944) 'The symptomatology and management of acute grief', *American Journal of Psychiatry* 101: 141–8.

Littlewood, J. (1992) *Aspects of Grief.* London: Routledge.

Maddison, D.C. *et al.* (1967) 'Factors affecting the outcome of conjugal bereavement', *British Journal of Psychiatry* 113: 1051–7.

Maxwell, N. (1996) 'Responses to loss and bereavement in HIV', *Professional Nurse* 12(1): 21–4.

Maxwell, R. (1984) 'Quality assessment in health', *British Medical Journal* i: 1470–2.

McGuiness, S. (1986) 'Death rites', *Nursing Times* March 19 28–31.

Parkes, C.M. (1986) *Bereavement: Studies of Grief in Adult Life.* London: Tavistock.

Parkes, C.M. (1987–8) 'Research – bereavement', *Omega* 18(4): 365–73.

Parkes, C.M. (1990) 'Risk factors in bereavement', *Psychiatric Annals* 20(6): 308–13.

Penson, J. (1990) *Bereavement – A Guide for Nurses.* London: Harper Row.

Pincus, L. (1976) *Death and the Family.* London: Faber & Faber.

Raphael, B. (1977) 'Preventive intervention with the recently bereaved', *Archives of Geriatric Psychiatry* 31(1): 450–4.

Raphael, B. (1985) *The Anatomy of Bereavement.* London: Hutchinson.

Schleifer, S. *et al.* (1983) 'Suppression of lymphocyte stimulation following bereavement', *Journal of the American Medical Association* 250: 374–7.

Sheldon, F. (1998) 'ABC of palliative care: bereavement', *British Medical Journal* 316: 456–8.

Walter, T. (1996) 'A new model of grief: bereavement and biography', *Mortality* 1: 7–25.

Walter, T. (1997) 'Letting go and keeping hold: a reply to Stroebe', *Mortality* 2(3): 263–6.

Worden, W. (1991) *Grief Counselling and Grief Therapy.* London: Routledge.

Wright, A. *et al.* (1988) *Matters of Death and Life.* London: Kings Fund Publications.

Practical matters following a death

8.1 Collecting the death certificate

The majority of hospitals have a bereavement office which deals with the legal and practical formalities following a patient's death. Bereaved relatives will usually need to return to the hospital to visit this office. In some facilities nursing staff will deal with these matters. Relatives should be given appropriate advice and directions at the time of the death.

Usually relatives are able to return to complete the formalities on the next working day after the death. In cases where burial is required within 24 hours for religious reasons, it will be necessary to arrange for a speedier completion of formalities. If possible, staff should try to arrange a definite appointment time for relatives to avoid unnecessary waiting.

Relatives *should not* be automatically informed that they will be able to collect the death certificate on their return. If the death is referred to the Coroner they will not be able to do so. This may not become clear until the patient's details are reviewed after the death.

Relatives of people with AIDS may be concerned about what is written on the death certificate. They should be able to talk to the doctor about their concerns. It may be possible to record the cause of death as the opportunistic infection which was the final cause of death.

Returning to complete legal formalities is a distressing time and relatives may need support. If they are unable to bring a friend or relative to support them, you may wish to consider arranging for other support within the hospital such as the hospital chaplain. Some ward staff arrange for the relatives to come back to the ward and then escort them to the bereavement office. This has the advantage of allowing relatives to meet a familiar member of staff and gives them further opportunity to discuss any aspects of the death which they still wish to raise. It is helpful to advise relatives to bring a suitcase or holdall to collect the patient's belongings.

If the patient had any money or valuables this is usually held centrally in the hospital's Cashiers Office. Property must only be handed over to people who are bona fide entitled to it. Proof of identity may be required and an indemnity form and receipt should be completed before property is handed over. In the case of very large sums of money Letters of Administration or Grant of Probate should be given as proof of identity.

When a patient dies outside the hospital setting the medical certificate of death will be obtained from the general practitioner. In cases of sudden death, the police may be involved.

Local bereavement office (for personal use)

8.2 Registering a death

Relatives are required to register a death within five days unless it has been reported to the Coroner. Under the Deaths Registration Act 1953 the following people are qualified to register the death. These are given in order of priority:

1 A relative of the deceased present at the death.
2 A relative of the deceased in attendance during the last illness.
3 A relative of the deceased residing in the district where the death occurred.
4 A person present at the death.
5 The 'occupier' (in patients with no next of kin this means a hospital manager).
6 Any 'inmate' aware of the death.
7 The person causing the disposal of the body.

It can be seen from this that the law usually demands that the death is registered by a relative. This can be tricky for cohabiting partners who may sometimes find that they have difficulties in registering the death, particularly where there is no will, and they may need to be assertive. Relatives should also be advised that registering the death is not a job that well meaning friends and neighbours can perform for them. They can give support by accompanying the relative, but the relative is usually required to attend in person. If there is any doubt about who should register the death or the information required the Registrar's department should be contacted by phone before arranging a visit. It would also be worthwhile to inform the Registrar's department if the person attending has any special needs such as a disability.

When registering a death relatives need to take the following items with them:

• Medical certificate of cause of death
• Medical card (if possible)

- Pension book (if in receipt of a war pension)
- Life insurance policies

They will also need to take the following information about the deceased:

- Date and place of death
- Last address
- Full name (and maiden name)
- Date and place of birth
- Last occupation
- State pension and benefits claimed
- Date of birth of widow/widower

The Registrar will supply a certificate for burial or cremation (known as the Green Form). The Registrar will also supply a copy of the Death Certificate on request. A fee is charged for this.

A certificate for Social Security purposes (Form BD8) is available on request. This is free of charge.

In some areas special arrangements are made at weekends for the Jewish and Muslim communities to register deaths in view of their need to bury their dead as quickly as possible. You should enquire locally to find out if these facilities are available.

Local Registrar's office (for personal use)

8.3 Post mortem examination and Coroner's enquiries

Coroners are obliged to investigate sudden unexpected deaths, any death where the cause is uncertain and unnatural deaths. The Coroner is required to investigate the circumstances of the death and to ascertain the identity of the person who died and the cause of death. For this reason, if a death is referred to the Coroner then formal identification of the body by the relatives will be necessary. This is usually arranged by the bereavement office. It is helpful if they can notify relatives of this duty in advance so that they are prepared for the event. It may be helpful if nursing staff advise relatives to telephone the office before attending.

More than one-third of deaths in England and Wales are referred to the Coroner. Deaths must be referred in the following circumstances:

1 The doctor has not been in attendance upon the patient during his or her last illness.
2 The doctor has not seen the patient during the 14 days immediately prior to death or seen the body after death.
3 The death may have been caused by an industrial disease.
4 Previous military service or War Pensioner.
5 Any sudden or unexplained death.
6 Any death in suspicious circumstances.
7 Any death which an accident may have caused or contributed towards. There is no time limit on this requirement.
8 Any death due to neglect, poisoning, misuse of drugs or abortion.
9 Any death in police custody or prison.
10 Any death which may be related to surgery or an anaesthetic. There is no formal time limit to this requirement.

Deaths may be reported to the Coroner if the hospital suspects that they come into one of the above categories. Normally this is established by the bereavement office. In addition, the Registrar may subsequently refer a death to a Coroner if not satisfied with the cause of death stated on the death certificate. Members of the public may report a death to the Coroner directly if they have reason for disquiet about the circumstances of the death. This can involve suspected unnatural deaths but can also involve cases where relatives or friends suspect negligence on the part of the medical practitioners.

When a death is reported to a Coroner four possible courses of action are available:

1 The Coroner will advise that an ordinary medical certificate of death may be issued by the doctor.
2 The Coroner will review the case but decide that no post mortem is necessary. He will then issue Pink Form A. This states that no post mortem examination is necessary and gives the cause of death.
3 The Coroner orders a post mortem examination. The pathologist then gives the cause of death in writing to the Coroner. If the death is natural the Coroner issues Pink Form B. This states the cause of death as established by the pathologist.
4 If death is found to be unnatural after a post mortem examination has taken place an inquest will be arranged. After this the Coroner will issue a certificate after inquest which will state the cause of death so that the death can be registered.

If a death is referred to the Coroner the bereavement office will usually explain to the relatives what is to happen. The relatives will then be required to contact the Coroner's office, where they will be informed about the investigations and advised about funeral arrangements. The Coroner may issue an Order for Burial (Form 101) or Certificate for Cremation (Form E) so that the funeral can take place. In cases where an inquest takes place the Coroner has the discretion to refuse cremation. The Coroner's office can also give relatives a letter confirming the death if this is needed for Social Security purposes.

Post mortem examinations

Medical post mortems can help doctors to understand more about the accuracy of diagnosis (Campbell 1997). If medical staff wish to carry out a post mortem examination and this has *not* been ordered by the Coroner they *must* ask the next of kin for permission to do so. Relatives have an absolute right to refuse permission. This should be explained to them and they should not be put under any undue pressure to give their consent. It may be possible to negotiate with relatives to carry out a limited post mortem to establish the cause of death.

Further reading

Campbell, N. (1977) 'Practice: post mortems: how and why they are carried out', *Nursing Times* 93(16): 52–4.

Local Coroner's office (for personal use)

8.4 Arranging a funeral

Arranging a funeral can be an added stress for bereaved relatives. Some relatives welcome the distraction of dealing with practical matters following a death but for many, these tasks are burdensome. The funeral is an important event bringing people together to remember the dead person. All too often funerals are mechanical and rushed and relatives too distressed to sit down and plan what they really want from the service. Nursing staff may help bereaved relatives with encouragement and advice. Some patients may want help in planning and recording their funeral wishes before their death.

Choosing a funeral director

Relatives can contact a funeral director as soon as they know of the death but should be advised not to make any definite funeral arrangements until they have found out whether or not the death is going to be referred to the Coroner. Coroner's investigations can delay the date of the funeral.

If relatives are unsure about contacting a funeral director they should be advised that the best method of choosing a funeral director is the personal recommendation of friends, relatives or neighbours. Nursing staff should not give advice on which particular firm to contact as this could be construed as a breach of their code of conduct.

Relatives can be advised to obtain written estimates before choosing a funeral director. There are a number of organizations representing funeral directors which each operate to their own code of practice.

The Funeral Standards Council represents the Co-Operative Funeral Society and a number of other independent firms. Their members subscribe to a 'Client's Pledge' and also belong to the Funeral Ombudsman Scheme which handles complaints against members. The Society of Allied and Independent Funeral Directors also belong to the Funeral Ombudsman Scheme.

Members of the National Association of Funeral Directors operate a code of practice, as do members of the Society of Allied and Independent Funeral Directors. Members of all three organizations are obliged to give their clients a price list and should not charge more than their written estimates without permission. Relatives can be advised to employ a funeral director who belongs to one of these organizations:

National Association of Funeral Directors
618 Warwick Road
Solihull
West Midlands. B91 1AA
Telephone: 0121 711 1343

Funeral Standards Council
30 North Road
Cardiff. CF1 3DY
Telephone: 02920 382046

Society of Allied and Independent Funeral Directors (SAIF)
Ferdinand Place
London. NW1 8EE
Telephone: 0207 267 6777

Internet: http://www.saif.org.uk

If a funeral director does not provide a satisfactory service or the prices charged appear to be unreasonable relatives can be advised to contact their local trading standards department. This will be listed in the telephone directory, usually under their local council offices.

The Citizen's Advice Bureau may also be able to help. Redress can also be sought from the Conciliation or Ombudsman Services of the organizations listed above.

The Association of Oddfellows publish an annual survey of funeral costs. This can give relatives an idea of whether an estimate is reasonable. Contact:

Oddfellows House
40 Fountain Street
Manchester. M2 2AB
Telephone: 0161 832 9361

Planning a funeral

Most funerals are not happy occasions. In spite of the grief we feel there should be opportunities for us to celebrate the life and achievements of the person who has died (Nuttall 1989). All too often, however, the funeral is reduced to a conveyor belt process, an expensive but empty ritual which leaves the bereaved with few positive memories.

In recent years there has been increasing criticism of the funeral industry (National Funerals College 1996). As a result there are now many organizations and resources which can help the bereaved to take charge of the funeral service and plan a fitting send off for the person they loved.

The dying person may wish to express his or her preferences regarding the funeral service. It is generally helpful if these wishes are recorded in writing. It is quite common for relatives to report conflicting verbal instructions from the deceased after the death and this can cause conflict within the family in the early days of bereavement.

It is generally up to the executor or personal representative of the deceased to decide on funeral arrangements. The National Funerals College recommend that people consider appointing a Funeral Guardian to carry out their wishes regarding their funeral. This person would be separate from the executor and would simply take responsibility for the funeral arrangements, relieving the burden on the executor. The executor does not have to follow the instructions left by the deceased about funeral arrangements. Sometimes families may choose to ignore the wishes of the deceased and the needs of the bereaved have to be balanced against the wishes of the deceased. A particularly common difficulty that occurs is when the dying person says that they want no funeral or memorial of any kind. This can be very unhelpful to the bereaved who may need the opportunity to grieve which a funeral can offer. The funeral also brings people together and can help to provide the bereaved with much needed social support.

Many funeral services are offered as a standard package. This package does not have to be accepted. Families can choose the venue for the service. This can be in a church or other place of worship or it could be in a local community centre with only the committal taking place in the cemetery or crematorium.

Families can plan the service that they want and make their own choice of readings, music and prayers. There are now several useful books containing suitable collections of readings and prayers (Bentley 1994; Sherrin 1996; Whitaker 1984).

If the family want a secular funeral the British Humanist Association runs a Helpline. They will be able to recommend someone locally to officiate at a secular funeral. Contact:

Telephone: 0990 168 122

The Dead Citizens Charter recommends that people should have the right to choose who conducts the funeral service and to have a service that

recounts the life and death of the person, recognising their uniqueness and the relationships that death has broken. (National Funerals College 1996)

Other choices that the family can be encouraged to make include where the body is to reside prior to the funeral, what the deceased should wear, whether the body should be embalmed and what type of coffin they require. This last item does not have to be obtained from the funeral director.

The following books can offer useful ideas and advice:

> Gill, Sue and Fox, John (19XX) *The Dead Good Funerals Book*. Engineers of the Imagination, Welfare State International.

Large parts of this book are reproduced on the London Association of Bereavement Services Website:

> http://www.bereavement.demon.co.uk/lbn/dg.html
>
> Hockey, J. (1992) *Making the Most of a Funeral*.
> Walter, T. (1991) *Funerals and How to Improve Them*.

Both these books are available from Cruse.

Useful organizations

National Funerals College
Braddan House
High Street
Duddington
Stamford
Lincs. PE9 3QE
Telephone: Unavailable

Aims to stimulate better funeral practice for the sake of the dead and the bereaved. It organizes training programmes and publishes the Dead Citizens Charter.

The Natural Death Centre
20 Heber Road
London. NW2 6AA
Telephone: 0208 208 2835

e-mail: rhino@dial.pipex.com
Internet: http://www.globalideasbank.org/naturaldeath.html

A non-profit making charitable project aiming to support those dying at home and their carers and to help them to arrange funerals. It has a more general aim of helping to improve the quality of dying. It has played a particularly important role in promoting and publicizing 'green' and 'DIY' funerals. Its website is an invaluable mine of useful information on death, dying and funerals. Publishes the *New Natural Death Handbook* which gives practical advice on death and funerals. A publications list is available. Also gives consumer advice by phone or letter on planning a funeral.

Cremation or burial?

Burial

Everyone of any religion has the right, in theory, to be buried in the churchyard of the parish in which they die. In practice many parish churchyards are full. It is possible to buy a licence known as a 'faculty' which reserves a space in a churchyard for future use. The executor will need to find out whether the deceased has already made this arrangement. It is also worth considering at the time of a funeral whether other members of the family will want to be buried next to the deceased in the future. In this case, the family will have to apply for a faculty to reserve the space.

Burial is also possible in cemeteries which are non-denominational and which may be either privately run or run by the local council. There are various categories of graves; the cheapest graves are without the right of exclusive burial (common graves). These are often used for DSS funerals and others may be buried in the same common grave (Drakeford 1998).

In most cemeteries it is possible to buy the right of exclusive burial *'in perpetuity'* while some grant exclusive rights for a specific number of years, for example, 50 years. Private 'lawn' graves can also be purchased, these are cheaper as they are on grass with just a simple headstone. Fees for burial in cemeteries can be obtained from the cemetery concerned. Fees for burial in churchyards can be obtained from the following address (ask for *A Guide to Church of England Fees*):

> **The Pastoral Department (General Section)**
> Church Commissioners
> 1 Millbank
> London. SW1P 3JZ

Cremation

In order to prevent cremation in cases where the cause of death is uncertain or suspicious there are strict rules about certification for cremation. Cremation must not occur if the deceased expressed an objection to it during their lifetime.

Three forms must be completed prior to cremation. Form A is an application for cremation which has to be completed by the executor or next of kin. Forms B and C are signed by two doctors; one must have attended the patient during their last illness and the other must see the body. Both doctors may charge a fee for signing the certificate. If the death is referred to the Coroner, these forms are not needed. The coroner will supply a certificate of cremation (Form E), which is free of charge.

Prior to cremation the medical referee appointed by the crematorium will scrutinize the certificates before signing Form F, which permits the cremation to go ahead. The medical referee's fees are included in the crematorium fee.

The fees for the cremation also include a fee for the use of the crematorium chapel. It is not necessary to have a funeral service at either a burial or cremation although most people find it beneficial. Crematoria are usually non-denominational so any type of religious or secular service can, in theory, be catered for. It is also quite possible to arrange for the service to take place elsewhere. Most crematoria work to a strict timetable of 15–20 minutes per service and if relatives want a longer service, extra time will have to be booked and paid for.

Following the service, it is possible for relatives to view the actual cremation if they wish to do so. This is a requirement in some religions.

It is most important for relatives to think about what they want done with the remains and make their wishes clear in advance. Routine procedure is for a crematorium to arrange for the ashes to be scattered in the garden of remembrance and a permanent memorial is not usually possible. Relatives may wish to consider whether they prefer to have the ashes buried or scattered at a particular site. Alternatively they may wish to keep the remains in an urn or casket, and the Natural Death Centre can advise on suppliers.

Following the cremation of a baby or young child, it is possible that little or no ashes will remain due to the cartilaginous nature of the bones.

Further advice on cremation can be obtained from:

The Cremation Society of Great Britain
Brecon House
Albion Place
Mainstone
Kent. ME14 5DZ
Telephone: 01622 688 292

The Federation of British Cremation Authorities
41 Salisbury Road
Carshalton
Surrey. SM5 3HA
Telephone: 0208 669 4521

DIY funerals

Some families may want to arrange their own funeral without the help of a funeral director. This can be a much cheaper option and can also give families a sense of control over saying goodbye to their loved one. The hospital mortuary may be persuaded to house the body until the time of the funeral, otherwise the family will have to arrange for care of the body at home in a cool place. DIY funerals will involve the family in organizing transport of the body, the funeral service and disposal of the body either by burial or cremation.

It is possible to bury a body on private land although extremely strict planning and public health rules apply. The most comprehensive information on 'DIY' funerals is available from the Natural Death Centre.

'Green' funerals

The past few years have seen an increased interest in 'green' funerals. These may include use of a biodegradable coffin or shroud and burial in a 'nature reserve' burial ground. The Natural Death Centre provide a guide to 'green' funerals and also run the Association of Nature Reserve Burial Grounds. Contact them for advice.

Burial at sea

It is possible to arrange burial at sea either through a funeral director or independently. There are only two places where sea burial is permitted: Newhaven and the Needles Spoil Ground to the west of the Isle of Wight. To arrange sea burial, it is necessary to obtain a Coroners Out of England Form and burial must be arranged through the Marine Environmental Protection Department at the Ministry of Agriculture, Fisheries and Food (Tel: 0171 238 5872).

An excellent guide to burial at sea is available on the Natural Death Centre website.

Memorials

Tangible memorials can play an important part in the grieving process (Clegg 1988). Advice about memorials and headstones can be obtained from the following organizations:

Memorial Advisory Bureau
139 Kensington High Street
London. W8 6SX
Telephone: 0207 937 0052

National Association of Memorial Masons
Crown Buildings
High Street
Aylesbury
Buckinghamshire. HP20 1SL
Telephone: 01296 434 750

Relatives may wish to consider ways of commemorating the deceased apart from the traditional headstone. Some relatives may wish to arrange for a specific bequest or donations to charity instead of floral tributes at the funeral. Relatives need to think early on about how they would like the deceased to be remembered. They may want to donate an item of equipment or furniture inscribed with the name of the deceased. Such bequests must be discussed with the organization concerned in advance. It is sensible to start collecting for the bequest as soon as possible as many people are most likely to donate at the time of the funeral service.

There are other ways that people can be remembered. Memorials by Artists has a nationwide register of artists making hand-carved memorials. Contact:

Memorials by Artists
Snape Priory
Saxmundham
Suffolk. IP17 1SA
Telephone: 01728 688 934

It is also possible to plant a tree or area of woodland as a memorial. Contact either of these organizations:

The National Memorial Arboretum
PO Box 10
Tisbury
Salisbury
Wiltshire. SP3 6TH

The Woodland Trust
Autumn Park
Dysart Road
Grantham
Lincolnshire. NG31 6LL

A simple, but good idea for creating a tangible memorial is to create a memorial box containing mementoes of the deceased. One idea is for mourners to contribute items to the box at the time of the funeral to be brought home afterwards. An alternative suggestion is a memorial book where mourners can record their memories of the deceased.

It is also possible to create a memorial on the Internet. You can create your own website or place an entry in either of the following:

The World Wide Cemetery

http://www.cemetery.org

This US organization charges for entries.

Virtual Memorial Garden

http://catless.ncl.ac.uk/vmg/vmg1.html

British run and free of charge.

Paying for a funeral

If relatives are likely to have difficulties paying for a funeral they should be advised to contact their local Social Security office. They may receive help from the Social Fund. This may be in the form of a grant or a loan which will have to be paid back out of the deceased patient's estate. Help with funeral costs is not generous (Drakeford 1998) and support and advocacy from a Welfare Rights adviser may be helpful at this time.

Advice may be obtained from the Benefits Enquiry Line:

Telephone: 0800 88 2200

The following booklets give helpful information:

'Help When Someone Dies' (DSS Leaflet, NI 19)
'What to Do After a Death' (DSS Leaflet D49)

It should be noted that anyone arranging a funeral will be liable for paying the bill. It is important for relatives to check where the money is coming from before making arrangements or they may end up with a bill that they cannot pay.

If there is no relative willing or able to pay for the funeral, the hospital, or in some cases the local authority, will be obliged to arrange to pay for the funeral. They will be able to make a claim on the deceased patient's estate to cover funeral costs.

When a patient dies in a hospital some distance from his or her home, the relatives may request that the hospital meets the cost of transporting the body back to the patient's home area. This may be met if the patient had been referred to a hospital distant from home. It will not normally be met if the patient was admitted to hospital when travelling or visiting the area.

Many local authorities provide a lower cost funeral service for local residents who would find the cost of a funeral difficult to meet. Your local council will be able to advise you on any services in your area.

Funerals abroad

Families with strong links overseas may wish to send the body of a deceased relative home for the funeral service.

Families wishing to export a body should be advised to contact a funeral director to make the necessary arrangements. Exporting a body can be an expensive undertaking and they should be advised to contact more than one funeral director for a quotation and to choose a funeral director who has considerable experience of the procedures. Further information can be obtained from The National Association of Funeral Directors.

Following the death the family must:

- Contact a funeral director
- Register the death

The family must inform the Registrar of their intention to export the body. The Registrar will supply them with a copy of the death certificate. There is a small charge for this.

The Registrar will also supply Form 104 which must be taken to the Coroner's office to obtain an 'Out of England' certificate allowing the body to leave the country.

The funeral director will usually arrange the necessary documentation. The following documents are required:

- Death certificate.
- Coroner's 'Out of England' certificate. (Coroners require four clear working days to complete their enquiries).
- Certificate of Embalming. All bodies must be embalmed to comply with airline and public health regulations.
- Certificate of freedom of infection: this is normally completed by the doctor who signed the death certificate. A fee may be charged.
- A declaration that the coffin contains only a body.

In addition the body must be hermetically sealed in a zinc-lined coffin and some countries also require a consular seal from the relevant embassy.

The funeral director should arrange all travel and transport. Costs will vary between different airlines so several quotes should be obtained. Some airlines may also be able to give advice and information about export of bodies.

If the death has been a subject of a Coroner's inquest the above procedure can be followed if death was from natural causes. However, if court proceedings have resulted from a death such as manslaughter or dangerous driving then the body cannot be repatriated until the court case is completed (Green and Green 1992).

References

Bentley, J. (1994) *Funerals Guide: Prayers, Hymns and Readings*. London: Hodder.

Clegg, F. (1988) 'Cremation, burial and memorials: the options and choices for bereaved people', *Bereavement Care* 7(2): 19–20.

Drakeford, M. (1998) 'Last rights? Funerals, poverty and social exclusion', *Journal of Social Policy* 27(4): 507–24.

Green, J. and Green, M. (1992) *Dealing with Death: Practices and Procedures*. London: Chapman and Hall.

National Funerals College (1996) The Dead Citizens Charter. Stamford, Lincs: National Funerals College.

Nuttal, D. (1989) 'The needs of the bereaved at the time of the funeral', *Bereavement Care* 3(3): 31–2.

Sherrin, N. (1996) *Remembrance*. London: Cruse.

Whitaker, A. (1984) *All In the End Is Harvest*. London: Cruse.

Part Four

CARING FOR THE RELIGIOUS NEEDS OF THE DYING

Meeting religious needs in the hospital setting

9.1 Nursing the dying of different faiths

In the final part of this book I will give information on a variety of different religious traditions and will outline their beliefs, particularly in respect of illness, suffering and death. These notes are not intended as a prescription for action, but as a resource to help the nurse to find out more about the patient's beliefs, primarily by talking to the patient directly.

It must always be remembered that whatever a patient's stated religion, their precise individual beliefs will be personal to them.

The UKCC Code of Conduct states that each registered nurse must:

> recognize and respect the uniqueness and dignity of each client and respond to their need for care irrespective of their ethnic origin, religious belief, personal attributes, the nature of their health problem or any other factor (UKCC 1992)

This chapter highlights some important issues which nurses should think about when planning individualized care of their patients.

Spiritual care

Recently, people have begun to make a distinction between spiritual and religious matters. Religion refers to a particular system of faith or worship whereas 'spiritual' is deemed to refer to a *personal search for meaning* which can be associated with secular beliefs such as humanism and atheism (Burnard 1988).

Dealing with the spiritual needs of dying patients means helping individuals to find meaning in suffering and responding to questions such as 'Why is this happening to me?' It also means responding to the painful feelings of sadness, anger and loss which may accompany such questions (Ainsworth-Smith and Speck 1982). Although the pastoral ministry of the chaplaincy and other religious leaders can be of enormous value, nurses may be the first to hear patients' spiritual concerns, as they often emerge during everyday encounters.

Saunders and Baines (1995) suggest that a feeling of meaninglessness is a form of spiritual pain. They say that everyone needs to look back at their life and

'feel that there was some sense in it' and reach out to 'something greater than themselves, a truth to which they can be committed.' (1995: 63)

Saunders and Baines emphasize the importance of simple presence; the need to be with the patient during their time of suffering. Hoy (1983) suggests that the dying patient needs a 'story hearer' who is willing to listen to their life story and who can help the patient to affirm the meaning and value of the life that they have lived. Listening and being with the patient are fundamental aspects of spiritual care.

Hoy (1983) stresses the need to maintain hope in the dying person. This will vary at different stages in the course of the illness. In the early stages of uncertainty a patient may still hope for a cure or remission and will need support to fight their illness. In the terminal phase hope may be for a peaceful death or for life after death. The importance of setting short term goals should not be forgotten. The patient can still have life to look forward to, however short, and should not be forced to wait only for death.

Ainsworth-Smith and Speck (1982) identify a hope for loving relationships as central to the concerns of the dying patient. This may involve being reconciled with the past. Since divorce and separation have become so commonplace, many people will have suffered domestic conflict and unhappiness and may have much 'unfinished business' to sort out in the last stages of their life.

Staff can help by encouraging open communication between families and avoiding collusion which keeps some family members in the dark (Maguire and Faulkner 1988). The chaplaincy can also offer support to patients and their families and friends at this time.

Caring for the dying patient demands that professional carers must also take stock of their own attitudes to death and their beliefs about the meaning of their own life (Ainsworth-Smith and Speck 1982).

Caring for dying patients can be a saddening experience but the courage and dignity with which many people face death can be a privilege to witness.

Religious traditions and beliefs

As well as providing spiritual care for patients we need to accommodate their particular religious beliefs and practices. Their religious beliefs may have an impact on activities of daily living such as dress, hygiene and diet. Their religious beliefs will also influence their views about health, illness, suffering and death. Religion may therefore affect both patients' treatment choices and their response to treatment.

Respect for a patient's religion means taking into account the way in which their religious beliefs influence the care and treatment which will be acceptable to them. It also means providing appropriate facilities to enable the patient to continue religious observances in the health care setting. These religious rituals may be of particular significance near to the time of death.

An understanding of the pattern of religious practices and beliefs in contemporary Britain can help nurses to address the religious needs of patients (Williams *et al.* 1998). Above all, Britain has become a country characterized by religious diversity. One reason for religious diversity is the fact that we now live in a multicultural society. Britain is ethnically and culturally diverse and with this diversity comes a multiplicity of religious traditions.

It is important not to confuse religious identity with ethnic identity (Weller 1997). Britain has become a religiously plural society over a long period of history and is now more religiously diverse than any other European country. All of the world's main religious traditions have a following in this country, although Christianity remains the 'official' and largest religious community. Our society is multicultural and multiethnic and so also are our religions. There are many 'Western' converts to 'Eastern' religions as well as the many African and Asian converts to Christianity. Most religious traditions are now ethnically diverse. In addition to members of the major world religions in the UK, there are also growing numbers of people who choose other forms of religious expression, belonging to new religious groups often described as *'sects'* or *'cults'* (Weller 1997).

Another important feature of contemporary British society is that it has become increasingly secular. Only 14 per cent of the population of Great Britain claim active membership of a Christian church, although this remains the religion of the majority of the population (Davie 1994).

This decline has been most marked in the Anglican church. In spite of this decline in religious observance, the majority of the population still claim to believe in God (Davie 1994). Thus for many people religion has become a private affair. People may hold personal religious convictions and engage in private prayer but have only tenuous connections with any religious organization. Births, marriages and funerals are still occasions when people turn to the church to provide the appropriate rituals and support, but for many people this is the only contact they have with their local church.

This has implications for nurses. The patient who is nominally Church of England may rarely set foot in a church but may have private religious convictions. In times of crisis such as a terminal illness, such people often turn to religion for explanation and comfort. This phenomenon has been described as the 'God of the gaps' (Abercrombie *et al.* 1970). The chaplaincy may have an important role to play with these patients.

The diversity of religious beliefs in contemporary Britain extends within the many religious groups in our society – within each group there may be varying traditions. To take Christianity as an example, there are many different Christian denominations. And even within one, such as Anglicanism, there are different traditions such as 'high church' and 'low church.' As for individuals there are, as we have seen, individuals who regularly attend church and those who never do.

These kinds of divisions and differences are present in all the world's religions to some extent. All individuals will vary both in terms of their particular beliefs and the strictness with which they adhere to them. Our best policy in understanding a patient's religious beliefs is to ask the patient.

9.2 The hospital chaplaincy

Most large hospitals have a hospital chaplaincy who provide pastoral support to patients in hospital and support for staff. The chaplaincy is usually a multi-faith department and its composition should reflect the religious composition of the surrounding community. Chaplains can help in the care of dying patients in the following ways.

Pastoral counselling by the chaplain with dying patients and their carers

Patients may often be concerned with religious and spiritual matters when faced with a life threatening illness. Patients who have not attended church recently may, however, be reticent about asking for the support of a chaplain. Nurses can help by offering the services of the chaplain to all patients and not just those who ask. The chaplain can be a useful person in whom the patient can confide their hopes and fears. The fact that they are not involved in delivering care can be reassuring to the patient. Chaplains should be involved sooner rather than later in the care of a patient where this is consistent with the patient's wishes. It is helpful if the chaplain is told precisely how much the patient has been told about their illness and prognosis. Once a chaplain has become involved with a patient they should be kept informed of any change, especially deterioration in the patient's condition. It can be very hurtful for a chaplain to discover the death of a patient only when he or she comes to the ward to visit.

Chaplains can also support the patient's family and friends. They can have particular value in offering continuity of support, especially when the patient moves between wards. Families may have to cope with a bewildering array of different staff and the chaplain can offer continuous support which will carry on after the death of the patient.

Staff support

Chaplains can also offer a listening ear to professional carers. Working with dying patients creates many stresses, and although ward staff usually support each other, sometimes a difficult situation with a patient can affect all staff with a sense of anxiety or a sense of sadness. It can be helpful to talk to someone outside the situation and a chaplain can sometimes perform this role in a more informal way than a professional counselling service.

Christian baptism/holy communion/time for confession

Dying people sometimes want to say and do things which they have chosen not to express all their lives. Some patients who have not been baptized seek baptism on their death bed (Eich 1987). This is an important spiritual and religious request which needs to be taken seriously. Where the desire for baptism is expressed to non-chaplaincy staff, you have a responsibility to ask the patient or their carers if they would like to see the chaplain to talk about the matter further. Where a positive response is received the chaplain should be contacted as soon as possible, and in larger hospitals an on-call service will be available.

Emergency baptism

1 Baptism should normally be carried out by the appropriate chaplain.
2 *In an emergency* when a chaplain cannot arrive in time, a member of staff may baptize the person as follows:

   (a) Collect some water in a bowl.
   (b) Dip your thumb into the water and make the sign of the cross on the person's forehead, while saying these words:

   (name of person) I BAPTIZE YOU IN THE NAME OF GOD, FATHER, SON AND HOLY SPIRIT. I SIGN YOU WITH THE SIGN OF THE CROSS, THE SIGN OF CHRIST. AMEN.

   The Lord's Prayer is now said,

   Our Father in heaven,
   hallowed be your name,
   your kingdom come,
   on earth as in heaven.
   Give us today our daily bread.
   Forgive us our sins,
   as we forgive those who sin against us.
   Lead us not into temptation,
   but deliver us from evil.
   For the kingdom, the power, and the glory are yours, now and forever. Amen.

3 *All baptisms* undertaken by staff must be recorded in the Baptism Register. The appropriate chaplain must be contacted as soon as possible so that this and any further pastoral work may be undertaken.
4 Baptism is essentially for those who are alive. The dead should not be baptized.

   You should contact one of your chaplains to discuss any further questions or reservations you may have about this.

Care of AIDS patients

Some people with HIV/AIDS feel that their illness has cut them off from the support and understanding of their church because of the stigma which it carries. Others put off approaching a church for fear of religious intolerance. The hospital chaplaincy can offer valuable support to AIDS patients with unfulfilled religious needs and can help a patient to make contact with a religious community. The Terence Higgins Trust also has an interfaith group which can put people with HIV/AIDS in touch with sympathetic clerics.

9.3 Spiritual healing

In some instances dying patients will want to turn to spiritual healing. It is important that patients have appropriate advice and support when choosing this option. Speck (1993) suggests that while spiritual healing can bring peace and comfort, it can also be a source of pressure, particularly if introduced by someone other than the patient. There is a danger that the patient might feel that if they do not recover physically this demonstrates their lack of faith. Speck (1993) suggests that this is a form of emotional blackmail.

If patients are considering spiritual healing the chaplaincy may be able to advise. Alternatively, advice on healing in a Christian context can be obtained from:

> **The Churches' Council for Health and Healing**
> St Marylebone Parish Church
> Marylebone Road
> London. NW1 5L7
> Telephone: 0207 486 9644

Alternatively, 'secular' healers can be contacted via the Healer Referral Service of the National Federation of Spiritual Healers:

> **NFSH**
> Old Farm Manor Studio
> Church Street
> Sunbury on Thames
> Middlesex. TW16 6RG
> Telephone: 0891 616 080

Ward communion

Some patients, especially Roman Catholics, may seek to have communion brought to them before they die. Again this is an important request which can meet spiritual and religious needs.

Formal confession/'reconciliation'

Most faiths say that after physical death has occurred the spirit of the person reviews the life that has been lived; rather like rewinding a video. Confession/'reconciliation' operates on the same principle, namely looking at who we are, what we have done, what we are sorry about and seek forgiveness for. It is an opportunity for some patients, most often Roman Catholics, to make their confession to God in the presence of the chaplain who mediates the forgiving love of God to the patient in the words of the Absolution.

References

Abercrombie N. *et al.* (1970) 'Superstition and religion: the God of the Gaps', in *A Sociological Year Book of Religion*. London: SCM.

Ainsworth-Smith, I. and Speck, P. (1982) *Letting Go: Caring for the Dying and Bereaved*. London: SPCK.

Burnard, P. (1988) 'The spiritual needs of atheists and agnostics', *Professional Nurse* December: 130–2.

Davie, G. (1994) *Religion in Britain Since 1945: Believing Without Belonging*. Oxford: Blackwell.

Eich, W. F. (1987) 'When is emergency baptism appropriate', *American Journal of Nursing* 87(12): 1680–1.

Hoy, T. (1983) 'Hospice chaplaincy in the caregiving team', in Corr, C.A. and Corr, D.M. (eds) *Hospice Care: Principles and Practice*. London: Faber and Faber.

Maguire, P. and Faulkner, A. (1988) 'Community with cancer patients: handling uncertainty collusion and denial', *British Medical Journal* 297(2): 972–4.

Saunders, C. and Baines, M. (1995) *Living with Dying*. Oxford: Oxford University Press.

Speck, P. (1993) Spiritual issues in palliative care, in *The Oxford Textbook of Palliative Medicine*. Oxford: Oxford University Press.

UKCC (1992) *Code of Professional Conduct for the Nurse, Midwife and Health Visitor*, 3rd edn. London: UKCC.

Weller, P. (1997) *Religions in the UK: A Multifaith Directory*. University of Derby in association with the Interfaith Network UK.

Williams A., Cooke, H. and May, C. (1998) *Sociology Nursing and Health*. Oxford: Butterworth–Heinemann.

Religious traditions and health care

This chapter offers information on a variety of different faiths. This is intended as background information. It should act as a starting point for individualized assessment of the patient. It should not act as a substitute for talking to patients and their families about the beliefs and preferences.

10.1 The Baha'i faith

Traditions and beliefs

The Baha'i faith began in Persia (now Iran) in the middle of the nineteenth century. It developed out of Shi'a Islam and in particular from an Islamic sect led by a religious leader known as the Bab (meaning gate or door). The Bab was executed for heresy in 1850 and following his death one of his followers, Baha 'u' Ullah (meaning 'glory of God') proclaimed himself leader. In 1867 Baha 'u' Ullah proclaimed himself a divine messenger ('*him whom God should manifest*'). Baha 'u' Ullah is seen as bringing divine revelation as foretold by former prophets. Baha'is believe that there has only ever been one God whom people have called by different names; Moses, Krishna, Zoroaster, Buddha, Christ and Mohammed are all believed to have been God's messengers. Baha 'u' Ullah was succeeded by first his son Abdu 'i' Baha and then his grandson, Shoghi Effendi. The writings of the four leaders, The Bab, Baha 'u' Ullah, Abdu 'l' Baha and Shoghi Effendi, make up the Baha'i scriptures (Hinnells 1996; Weller 1997).

Following the death of Shoghi Effendi, a 'Universal House of Justice' was founded in Israel and this is now the governing body of the Baha'is.

Baha'is believe that the future of the world lies in creating a single world order establishing the unity of mankind (Weller 1997). Baha'is believe in world peace and are in favour of equality of race, gender and class. Baha'is also believe in the unity of science and religion and promote the importance of education and knowledge.

Social and charitable service are also an important part of the Baha'i faith.

Every Baha'i over the age of 15 must recite three prayers each day (known as the '*salat*' as in Islam). Ritual washing precedes these prayers. When praying, Baha'is must face the burial place of Baha 'u' Ullah which is at Bahji in Akka, Israel. (This is in a south-easterly direction. A map of the hospital marked with points of the compass is useful as an aid.) Baha'is are also expected to read from the scriptures each day (Weller 1997).

The Baha'i year consists of 19 months each of 19 days beginning on the Spring equinox. Baha'is are expected to attend religious festivals known as the Nineteen Day Feasts at the beginning of each Baha'i month. Baha'is are also encouraged to make a pilgrimage to one of the Baha'i holy sites.

The Baha'i faith is organized through 'Spiritual Assemblies'. These are found at both local and national levels. Assemblies are elected bodies who make decisions about their community and arrange meetings. Baha'is are encouraged to move to parts of the world where there are no Baha'is to spread the faith. There are currently 6,000 Baha'is in Britain connected to 380 local groups or assemblies (Weller 1997). Some Baha'is in Britain originate from Iran, but many are British converts. The Baha'i faith first came to Britain in 1899. There are approximately six million Baha'is worldwide and the religion is rapidly growing.

Daily living, health and healing

There are no dietary proscriptions, but Baha'is are encouraged to become vegetarians. There is a period of fasting in the Baha'i month of Ala (2–21 March). During this period, Baha'is are expected to fast from sunrise to sunset. Children, the elderly, invalids and pregnant or nursing mothers are exempt from fasting.

Abstention from alcohol and other harmful or addictive drugs is required. Alcohol must not be used in any form and this includes as a flavouring in cooking. Narcotics are permitted where they are part of bona fide medical treatment (National Spiritual Assembly of the Baha'is 1993). Smoking is strongly discouraged.

There is no objection to blood transfusion and organ donation is regarded as praiseworthy.

Baha'is in hospital will appreciate facilities for prayer. This may include a quiet area for prayer and appropriate washing facilities (National Spiritual Assembly of the Baha'is 1993).

Death and dying

There is no specific ritual following a death and routine Last Offices would be appropriate. Baha'is believe that the body should be treated with respect. Cremation is not permitted and burial should take place as near as possible to the place of death and certainly not more than one hour's journey away.

Post mortem is permitted providing these stipulations are met (National Spiritual Assembly of the Baha'is 1993).

Baha'is are buried with their feet facing the tomb of Baha 'u' Ullah.

National contacts

National Baha'i Community of the United Kingdom
27 Rutland Gate
London. SW7 1PD
Telephone: 0207 584 2566

Baha'i Publishing Trust
6 Mount Pleasant
Oakham
Leicester
Telephone: 01572 722780

Local group (for personal use)

References and further reading

Hinnells, J. (1996) *A Handbook of Living Religions,* 2nd edn. Oxford: Blackwells.
National Spiritual Assembly of the Baha'is (1993) *Members of the Baha'i Faith as Hospital Patients: Some Notes for Nurses, Doctors and Healthcare Workers.*
New Encyclopedia Britannica (1989) 15th edn. 'Baha'i Faith'. Chicago: Encyclopedia Britannica, pp. 797–8.
Smart, N. (1992) *The World's Religions.* Cambridge: Cambridge University Press.
Weller, P. (1997) *Religions in the UK: A Multifaith Directory,* 2nd edn. University of Derby in Association with the Interfaith Network UK.

Internet resources

http: //www.northill.demon.co.uk/bahai/index.htm

A short introduction to the Baha'is based on a book of the same name.

http: //www.fragrant.demon.co.uk/warwick.html

The home pages of the Warwick Assembly of the Baha'is.

10.2 Buddhism

Traditions and beliefs

Buddhists follow the teachings of Gautama Buddha. Gautama Buddha lived in what is now Nepal in the fifth century BC. He is accepted as a great teacher and is not believed to have had divine status. Buddhists believe in the four noble truths.

1 *Dukka* – all life is characterized by *dukka* (suffering or unsatisfactoriness).
2 *Samudaya* – the origin of *dukka* is desire and selfishness.
3 *Nirodha* – *dukka* (suffering) can be overcome by the cessation of desire and is known as *nibbana* (self annihilation).
4 *Majjhima Patipada* (The Middle Way or Eightfold Path). The eightfold path of enlightenment will overcome *dukka*. This comprises correct vision, right thoughts, right speech, right conduct, right livelihood, right effort, right mindfulness and right meditation.

There are two main traditions in Buddhism and it is important to identify which tradition an individual belongs to: the Theravada tradition, originating in Sri Lanka, Burma, Laos, Cambodia and Vietnam (Southern Transmission) and the Malayan tradition, originating in China, Japan, Korea and Tibet (Northern Transmission). There are approximately 130,000 Buddhists in this country. Many minority ethnic communities of Chinese and Vietnamese origins follow Buddhist beliefs and practices. There are also many native British converts to Buddhism. There are an estimated 328 million Buddhists worldwide.

Daily living, health and healing

The Five Precepts (Panci Silani) are the rules for living for lay Buddhists. These are the basis of 'right action' one of the aspects of the Eightfold Path. The five precepts involve refraining from harming living beings and from stealing, sexual misconduct, harmful speech, drink or drugs. Buddhists will also practise meditation (Weller 1997).

Buddhists emphasize the avoidance of killing and therefore most Buddhists are vegetarians or vegans. Chinese Buddhists also avoid the consumption of garlic and onions: they are believed to heat the blood and make meditation difficult. Many Buddhists also abstain from alcohol. Buddhist patients in hospital may appreciate the opportunity for peace and quiet to facilitate meditation.

Death and dying

Buddhists believe that the state of mind at death will influence what happens to the individual after death. Buddhists are expected to meditate at the time of death and may refuse drugs, particularly analgesics, which will affect their mental clarity at the moment of death. It is therefore important to discuss the effects of drugs with Buddhist patients. Buddhist patients who are dying may benefit from the presence of a

Buddhist monk or member of a local Buddhist organization. Some Buddhists will take comfort from a statue or picture of the Buddha or a revered Buddhist teacher. Copies of Buddhist sacred writings in book form or on audiotape may also be required. Sometimes Buddhists may wish to light a candle or burn incense when meditating (Buddhist Hospice Trust (undated)).

Rites and practices after death will depend on the ethnic origin of the patient. For most Buddhist patients routine Last Offices will be appropriate but relatives should be contacted for advice, as some Buddhist sects have strong views on how the body should be treated.

There is usually no religious objection to post mortems or organ donation. Cremation is usual, with subsequent burial of the ashes.

National contacts

Buddhist Society
58 Eccleston Square
London. SW1V 1PH
Telephone: 0207 834 5858

Buddhist Hospice Trust
Flat 1, Laural House
Trafalgar Road
Newport
Isle of Wight. PO30 1QN
Telephone: 01983 526 945

Edinburgh Buddhist Centre
55a Grange Road
Edinburgh
Lothian. EH9 1TX

Friends of the Western Buddhist Order
c/o London Buddhist Centre
51 Roman Road
Bethnal Green
London. E2
Telephone: 0207 981 1225

Samye Ling Tibetan Centre (Rokpa Trust)
Eskdalemuir
Langholm
Dumfries and Galloway. DG13 0QL

Internet resources

Samye Ling Tibetan Centre
http://www.samye.org

Local contacts (for personal use)

References and further reading

Buddhist Hospice Trust (Undated). *Spiritual Needs of Seriously Ill and Dying Buddhists.*

Hardacre, H. (1994) 'Response of Buddhism and Shinto to the issue of brain death and organ transplant', *Cambridge Quarterly of Healthcare Ethics*, 3: 585–601.

Irish, D. *et al.* (1990) *Ethnic Variations in Dying, Death and Grief.* Washington: Taylor and Francis.

Keene, M. (1993) *Seekers After Truth: Hinduism, Buddhism, Sikhism.* Cambridge: Cambridge University Press.

Bukkyo Dendo Kyokai (1993) *The Teaching of Buddha.* Tokyo: Society for the Promotion of Buddhism

Sullivan, L.E. (1989) *Healing and Restoring: Health and Medicine in the World's Religious Traditions.* New York: Macmillan.

Weller, P. (1997) *Religions in the UK: A Multifaith Directory*, 2nd edn. University of Derby in association with The Interfaith Network UK.

Internet resources

http: //www.fwbo.org/buddhism.html.
A site on Buddhism by the Friends of the Western Buddhist Order.

10.3 Christianity

Traditions and beliefs

All Christian groups believe in the teachings of Jesus of Nazareth and almost all believe that God became man on earth in the person of Jesus Christ. Most Christians believe that Jesus rose from the dead and ascended to heaven and that his death and resurrection have redeemed mankind from sin.

There are three major groups within the Christian Church: the Orthodox Church, the Protestant Churches and the Roman Catholic Church. There are also a large number of sectarian Christian groups which can be regarded as offshoots from the Protestant Churches.

There are approximately 40 million members of Christian churches in this country although only 7 million of these are regular churchgoers. Christianity is the largest and longest established UK religion (Weller 1997). In this section I will consider some of the major Christian groupings.

The Orthodox Church

Traditions and beliefs

The Orthodox Churches are the Churches of Greece, Eastern Europe and North Africa and are to be found in the UK in areas with migrant populations from these areas. Orthodoxy claims to represent a more original form of Christianity than Roman Catholicism or Protestantism and traces its roots back to before the division of Eastern and Western Christianity (Weller 1997).

The Orthodox Church gives central importance to the Holy Trinity and believes that the Spirit of God proceeds from God the Father alone and not from God the Son as stated in the Catholic Nicene Creed. This difference of opinion is known as the 'filioque controversy' and is the major theological difference between Orthodox and other Christian churches.

The main Orthodox Churches in this country are the Greek and Russian Orthodox Churches. There are four Patriarchates in the Orthodox Church who claim direct descent of authority from the apostles. These are the Patriarchates of Alexandra, Antioch, Constantinople and Jerusalem. In addition there are a large number of 'autocephalic' (literally 'himself the head', meaning nationally independent) churches, such as the Serbian, Byelorussian and Ukrainian Autocephalic Churches. There are also a growing number of Oriental Orthodox Churches in Britain, in particular the Armenian, Coptic and Ethiopian Churches. There is a small British Orthodox community (The Orthodox Church of the British Isles).

Not all Orthodox Churches are in communion with each other and when a patient states that their Christian denomination is Orthodox they should be asked to which jurisdiction they belong. For example, the Greek and Russian Orthodox Churches are not in communion with the Coptic and Serbian Churches.

Daily living, health and healing

There are no special requirements regarding the treatment of Orthodox patients in hospital, although many would wish to be visited by a priest. The Orthodox attitude to illness and suffering means that some Orthodox patients may be reluctant to take analgesia (Harakas 1986; Nikodemus Orthodox Publication Society 1986).

Death and dying

It is usual practice in the Orthodox Church to anoint for healing anyone who is sick and the patient may also wish to take the Sacrament. When death is imminent, a priest should be present to say committal prayers.

The priest should also be present after death to carry out religious observances (in the Greek Orthodox Church this is the Trisaghion Service) as
soon as the patient has died. Obviously it is important to inform the
Orthodox priest if any Orthodox patient is seriously ill.

Cremation is not permissible.

National contacts

Armenian Apostolic Oriental Orthodox Council
St Peter's Church
Cranley Gardens
London. SW7 3BB
Telephone: 0207 937 0152

Byelorussian Autocephalic Orthodox Church
Mother of God Zyrovicy Church
Chapel Road
Rainsborough
Prestwich
Manchester. M22 4JW
Telephone: 0161 740 8330

Coptic Orthodox Church
Allen Street
London. W8 6VX
Telephone: 0207 937 5782

Ethiopian Orthodox Church
253 Ladbroke Grove
London. W10 6HF
Telephone: 0208 960 3848

Greek Orthodox Archdiocese of Thyateira and Great Britain
Thyateira House
5 Craven Hill
London. W2 3ED
Telephone: 0207 723 4787

The Orthodox Church of the British Isles
The Stable Court
Castle Howard
York. YO6 7DA
Telephone: 0165 384 350

Orthodox Church in Wales
(Yr Eglwys Uniongred yug Nghymru)
11 Manod Road
Blaenau Festiniog
Gwynnedd. LL41 4DE

Russian Orthodox Church
All Saints
67 Ennismore Gardens
London. SW7 1NH
Telephone: 01234 354 374

Syrian Orthodox Church's Council (UK)
Antaccia
77 Exeter Road
London. N14 5JU
Telephone: 0208 368 8447

Ukrainian Autocephalous Orthodox Church
1A Newton Avenue
Acton
London. W3 8AJ
Telephone: 0208 992 4689

Local contacts (for personal use)

Roman Catholicism

Traditions and beliefs

The Roman Catholic Church view the Bishop of Rome (The Pope) as the head of the Church. They believe in the Apostolic succession of the Pope, i.e. that the Pope is the lawful successor to Peter the Apostle appointed by Jesus to be head of his Church. The Pope is therefore believed to be infallible since his is invested with Christ's authority.

The Church is centrally organized in a hierarchy of cardinals, bishops and priests. Important aspects of Catholic worship are Mass (Holy Communion) and confession. There are approximately 5 million Catholics in Britain (Weller 1997).

Daily living, health and healing

There is a Roman Catholic chaplaincy team in most hospitals and Catholic patients should be asked whether they would like to see a chaplain while they are in hospital.

Catholic patients may wish to receive Holy Communion while they are in-patients or to attend Sunday Mass. Many Catholics will abstain from eating meat on Fridays.

Death and dying

Any sick or dying patient may wish to receive the anointing of the sick (if desired) and the chaplain should be contacted if required. After death the family may wish to say prayers with the chaplain.

National contacts

Roman Catholic Church in England and Wales
39 Eccleston Square
London. SW1V 1PD
Telephone: 0207 233 8196

Roman Catholic Church in Scotland
Central Hall
West Toll Cross
Edinburgh
Lothian. EH3 9BP
Telephone: 0131 229 7937

Local contacts (for personal use)

Most hospitals will have a Roman Catholic chaplain who can be contacted via the hospital switchboard.

Protestant Churches

There are a wide variety of Protestant Churches, denominations and sectarian groups. The main groups will be briefly covered in this section.

The Anglican Church

The Anglican Church is the 'official' Church in this country. There are four autonomous Anglican churches: The Church of England, The Scottish Episcopal Church, the Church of Wales and the Church of Ireland. It was founded during the Reformation in 1534 and its main organizational difference from the Catholic Church is that it does not acknowledge the Pope as its head. The monarch is the supreme Governor of the Church of England while its spiritual leader is the Archbishop of Canterbury (Weller 1997).

Daily living, health and healing

Anglican patients should be asked whether they would wish to see a hospital chaplain during their stay.

Death and dying

The Anglican chaplain should be called if required to support the patient and relatives.

Local contacts (for personal use)

The Free Churches

The Free Church Council was founded in 1940 to represent several different Protestant Churches. Members of the following Churches could appropriately be visited by a Free Church chaplain:

- The Baptist Union of Great Britain and Ireland
- Congregational Federation
- Countess of Huntingdon's Connexion
- Independent Methodist Churches
- The Methodist Church

- The Moravian Church
- The Presbyterian Church
- The Salvation Army
- The United Reformed Church
- The New Testament Church of God
- The Fellowship of Churches of Christ
- The Free Church of England
- The Wesleyan Reform Union
- The United Free Church of Scotland

Daily living, health and healing

The Free Churches are variants of Protestant Christianity. There may be slight variations in their beliefs but in general there will be no special religious requirements in hospital other than to be visited by a chaplain if requested (Sampson 1982).

The United Reformed Church produce a number of helpful booklets from a broadly Christian viewpoint on illness, grief and loss. Contact:

> **Health and Healing Committee**
> The United Reformed Church
> 86 Tavistock Place
> London. WC1H 9RT
> Telephone: 0207 916 2020

Death and dying

There are no special religious requirements but the patient and relatives may appreciate the support of a chaplain. Routine Last Offices are appropriate.

Other Christian groups

Brethren

The Brethren movement was founded in the nineteenth century. The Brethren are local independent congregations and include those described as 'Plymouth' or 'Exclusive' Brethren. They believe that they practise a more truly original pattern of Christianity.

Daily living, health and healing

Some Brethren are reluctant to mix with non-Brethren. They may be reluctant to talk to other patients and even, on occasions, ward staff. They will value privacy and may also wish their own meals to be brought in for them. Some Brethren will wish to wear an article of clothing at all times even when bathing (Sampson 1982).

Death and dying

The dying Brethren patient would wish to be visited by religious representatives from his/her own congregation. Some may be willing to see the Free Church chaplain.

Contact

Contact should be through the patient's friends and family. There are many different independent congregations of Brethren (953 nationally).

Christian Scientists

The Church of Christ, Scientist was founded by Mary Baker Eddy in the nineteenth century. Christian scientists believe that disease and suffering can be healed by prayer alone. Mary Baker Eddy published *Science and Health with Key to the Scriptures* which supplements the Bible in Christian Science worship and teaching (Weller 1997). There are 220 Christian Science congregations in Britain.

Daily living, health and healing

Many Christian Scientists would not accept conventional medical treatment and therefore would not seek medical help. Exceptions to this are medical care during pregnancy and childbirth and medical care for children. Christian Scientists will seek medical help for their children as this is required of them under the law (The Children and Young Persons Act 1935 states that a doctor must be called to a child in case of illness). Christian Scientists may also agree to have bones set as they regard this as a mechanical procedure (Christian Science Publishing Society 1974; Schoepflin 1986).

Christian Scientists are most likely to be in hospital as a result of trauma and may wish to be removed to a Christian Science nursing home as soon as is practicable. The Church of Christ Scientist claims that Christian Scientists are under no pressure to refuse medical treatment and are free to make up their own mind according to their conscience. Christian Scientists will comply with all necessary public health regulations such as notification of infections etc. As with all cases of refusal of life saving treatment, staff must ascertain that refusal is valid (*Re T* 1992).

The Christian Scientist patient is expected to refrain from tobacco and alcohol. There are no special dietary restrictions.

Death and dying

There are no special last rites and routine Last Offices would be appropriate. The body of a female should be handled by female staff. Post mortems are refused unless legally required.

National contacts

Church of Christ, Scientist
108 Palace Gardens
London. W8 4RT
Telephone: 0207 221 5650

Church of Christ Scientist
Christian Science Committee on Publication
2 Elysium Gate
126 New Kings Road
London. SW6 4LZ
Telephone: 0207 371 0060

Local contacts (for personal use)

The Church of Jesus Christ of Latter Day Saints (Mormon)

The Mormon Church was founded by Joseph Smith in the United States. Mormons believe that Joseph Smith found an ancient scripture hidden in a hill near New York. They believe that the ancient Israelites were the ancestors of the American Indians and that their scriptures were written on gold plates which were rediscovered by Joseph Smith and translated into English by the gift of God. These became the 'Book of the Mormon' which is the Mormons' main scripture alongside the Bible. Mormons also believe that Jesus visited America after his Ascension (Weller 1997).

Daily living, health and healing

Mormon patients may wish to pray regularly during the day and would wish to have access to a copy of the Book of the Mormon as well as the Bible.

Mormons wear a special undergarment which is considered sacrosanct. This is worn at all times and is only removed for hygiene purposes, although it would be permissible to remove it when the patient attends theatre (Sampson 1982).

Mormons refrain from drinking tea, coffee, alcohol and cola drinks. They also refrain from smoking. *All* stimulants are forbidden and some Mormons will refuse all hot drinks. Prescribed drugs may be taken under medical direction. Mormons are required to fast for 24 hours every month but this would be waived under medical direction (Bush 1986).

Mormons would wish to be visited by a local church leader who may wish to give 'priesthood blessings' to the sick.

Death and dying

There are no special rituals for the dying but a visit from a local church leader would be appreciated. There is no special requirement for Last Offices except that the patient's 'sacred undergarment' be replaced on the body.

National contacts

International Headquarters:

> **The Church of Jesus Christ of Latter Day Saints**
> Public Communications Department
> 50 East North Temple Street
> Salt Lake City
> Utah. 84150 USA

National contact:

> **The Church of Jesus Christ of Latter Day Saints**
> 751 Warwick Road
> Solihull
> West Midlands. B91 3DQ
> Telephone: 0121 709 2244

Local contacts (for personal use)

Jehovah's Witnesses

The Jehovah's Witness movement was founded in the nineteenth century in North America by Charles Taze Russell. Russell founded the Zion's Watch Tower Society to disseminate Bible truths. The Watch Tower Society now distributes Jehovah's Witness Literature throughout the world. Jehovah's Witnesses have their own translation of the Bible, in which God is called Jehovah. (Beckford 1975; Weller 1997).

Local congregations of Jehovah's Witnesses meet in Kingdom Halls and are organized by a group of elders. There is a strong emphasis on Bible study and doorstep evangelism.

Jehovah's Witnesses regard the present day as a time of Satan and look forward to the coming of Armageddon (Schmalz 1994). They believe that Jehovah rules heaven alongside Jesus Christ and 144,000 chosen people who once lived on earth. They believe that the coming of Jehovah's Kingdom on Earth is imminent.

Jehovah's Witnesses are not supposed to hold political office, vote, join the armed forces or salute the flag. They believe that they owe their allegiance to divine, rather than secular authority. Most Witnesses do not celebrate Christmas or birthdays (Cumberland 1986).

Daily living, health and healing

Jehovah's Witnesses have no special requirement for care other than their well known prohibition on the use of blood transfusions. Blood transfusions were officially banned by the Witnesses in 1945 and this stance was linked to their position as conscientious objectors in the Second World War (Singelenberg 1990). Prior to this time Jehovah's Witnesses discouraged immunization but there is now no religious objection to immunization among Witnesses (Cumberland 1986; Singelenberg 1990).

The Jehovah's Witness blood transfusion taboo is based mainly on passages from Leviticus which indicate substances to be avoided. These passages lay down Jewish dietary requirements. Witnesses do not, however, require Kosher food but they do avoid foodstuffs made exclusively of blood, such as black pudding.

Jehovah's Witnesses now also employ an array of secular arguments against blood transfusion emphasizing the dangers and the risk of blood-borne infection (Watch Tower 1990). Jehovah's Witness literature also emphasizes the fact that alternatives to blood transfusion are available (Watch Tower 1996).

The religious position on blood transfusions has hardened over the past twenty years and autologous blood transfusions are now also forbidden (Cumberland 1986). Accepting blood fractions such as immunoglobulin is considered to be a matter of individual conscience (Watch Tower 1996). Usually only blood substitutes such as plasma expanders and iron supplements will be acceptable.

The Jehovah's Witness in hospital will want to be reassured that they will not be given blood or blood products. On admission to hospital, staff may require Jehovah's Witnesses to indicate their wish to refuse blood on a standard form. This form should forcefully bring to the patient's attention the possible consequences of refusal (*Re T* 1992).

In all life threatening situations where a medical treatment is refused, staff have a duty to ensure that refusal is valid, that the patient fully understands the consequences of refusal and that their decision is not made under duress or undue influence (*Re T* 1992). In the case of children, legal advice should always be obtained.

Many Jehovah's Witnesses carry Medical Alert cards signed and witnessed by two other Jehovah's Witnesses indicating their intention to refuse blood transfusion. These cards carry the same problem of all advance directives that they must be valid and applicable to existing circumstances (see Chapter 3). If in any doubt, legal advice should be obtained (*Re T* 1992). It should also be noted that relatives cannot give or refuse consent to treatment on a patient's behalf.

Non-Witness relatives of Jehovah's Witnesses can sometimes feel isolated and may need support, especially if their relative is refusing a blood transfusion. It is important that staff ensure that patients continue to have access to their non-Witness relatives and friends.

Death and dying

Jehovah's Witnesses will want to be visited by their congregation. Routine Last Offices are appropriate.

Some Jehovah's Witnesses will consent to organ donation but others will refuse. Jehovah's Witnesses usually refuse post mortem dissection unless this is required by the coroner (Watch Tower 1996).

There are no special funeral rites and either burial or cremation is permitted.

National contact

Watch Tower Society
The Ridgeway
London. NW7 1RN
Telephone: 0208 906 2211

Local contacts (for personal use)

The Religious Society of Friends (Quakers)

The Society of Friends was founded by George Fox in the seventeenth century. Quakers believe that everyone may have a direct experience of God and that there is 'that of God in everyone'. Quakers do not have a paid ministry and hold 'meetings for worship' which largely involve silent meditation. Meetings are organized by a 'clerk'. Quakers have strong beliefs in pacifism and the importance of social service (Gillman 1988).

Daily living, health and healing

Quakers may be visited by the local Pastoral Care Team (called 'Overseers') while in hospital. When caring for a Quaker it would be helpful to ask the patient the name of the clerk of the Meeting which they attend and what contact the patient would like to be made. Most Quakers would be happy to be visited by a hospital chaplain.

Death and dying

Quakers are explicitly reminded to prepare for death and most would prefer to be told the truth sooner rather than later. Members of the Pastoral Care Team will visit and may wish to hold Meetings for Worship at the bedside of a Quaker patient. A quiet and peaceful area of the ward would be appreciated for this; as meetings are largely silent, they would not be disruptive.

There are no special last rites and routine Last Offices would be appropriate (Pym 1992).

National contact

Quaker Home Service
Friends House
Euston Road
London. NW1 2BJ
Telephone: 0207 387 3601

Local contacts (for personal use)

Seventh Day Adventists

Seventh Day Adventism was founded in North America in the nineteenth century by Ellen Gould White. A key belief is that the Sabbath should be celebrated on the seventh day (Saturday). Seventh Day Adventists share many beliefs with other Christian Evangelical groups. The Seventh Day Adventist movement is particularly popular among the Afro Caribbean Community (Sampson 1982; Weller 1997).

Daily living, health and healing

Many Seventh Day Adventists are lacto vegetarians, a few being vegan. Some, however, eat certain flesh foods, avoiding pork, shellfish and other articles which are described as unsuitable in the biblical record of Leviticus.

All Seventh Day Adventists abstain from the use of tobacco and alcoholic drinks and many avoid tea, coffee and other caffeinated drinks (Numbers and Amundsen 1986).

Death and dying

There are no special last rites but all Seventh Day Adventists will wish to be ministered to by their own pastor prior to death.

National contact

Seventh Day Adventist Church
Stanborough Park
Watford. WD2 6JP
Telephone: 01923 672 251

Local contacts (for personal use)

Spiritualism

Spiritualists believe that the soul survives death and can communicate with loved ones on earth through the use of mediums (Sampson 1982).

Daily living, health and healing

There are no special requirements, although some spiritualists may be vegetarian.

Dying and death

The dying patient will appreciate a visit from the local spiritualist minister. There are no special requirements for Last Offices. Some spiritualists will be opposed to cremation (Sampson 1982).

References and further reading

Beckford, J. (1975) *The Trumpet of Prophecy: A Sociological Study of Jehovah's Witnesses*. Oxford: Basil Blackwell.

Brierley, P. (1996/7) *UK Christian Handbook*. London: Christian Research Association.

Bush, L.E. (1986) 'The Mormon Tradition', in Numbers, R. and Amundsen, D. (eds) *Caring and Curing: Health and Medicine in the Western Religious Traditions*. New York: Macmillan.

Christian Science Publishing Society (1974) *Questions and Answers on Christian Science*. Boston: Christian Science Publishing Society.

Cross, F.L. and Livingstone, E.A. (eds) (1997) *Oxford Dictionary of the Christian Church*, 3rd edn. Oxford: Oxford University Press.

Cumberland, W.H. (1986) 'The Jehovah's Witness tradition', in Numbers, R. and Amundsen, D. (eds) *Caring and Curing: Health and Medicine in the Western Religious Traditions*. New York: Macmillan.

Gillman, H. (1988) *A Light is Shining: An Introduction to the Quakers*. London: Quaker Home Service.

Harakas, S. (1986) 'The Eastern Orthodox tradition', in Numbers, R. and Amundsen, D. (eds) *Caring and Curing: Health and Medicine in the Western Religious Traditions*. New York: Macmillan.

Hinnells, J. (1996) *A New Handbook of Living Religions*. Oxford: Blackwells.

Irish, D. *et al.* (1990) *Ethnic Variations in Dying, Death and Grief*. Washington: Taylor and Francis.

Nikodemos Orthodox Publication Society (1986) *The Teachings of the Holy Fathers on Illness*. Redding, California: Nikodemus Orthodox Publication Society.

Numbers, R. and Amundsen, D. (1986) *Curing and Curing: Health and Medicine in the Western Religious Traditions*. New York: Macmillan.

Pym, J. (1992) *Quakers and Death*. London: Quaker Home Service.

Re T (1992) (Refusal of Medical Treatment). Independent Court of Appeal, 30 July 1992.

Sampson, A.C. (1982) *The Neglected Ethic: Religious and Cultural Factors in the Care of Patients*. London: McGraw Hill.

Schoepflin, R. (1986) 'The Christian Science tradition', in Numbers, R. and Amundsen, D. (eds) *Caring and Curing: Health and Medicine in the Western Religious Traditions*. New York: Macmillan.

Schmalz, M. (1994) 'When Festinger fails: prophecy and Watch Tower', *Religion* 24: 293–308.

Singelenberg, R (1990) 'The blood transfusion taboo of Jehovah's Witnesses: origin, development and function of a controversial doctrine', *Social Science and Medicine* 31(4): 515–23.

Watch Tower (1990) *How Blood Can Save Your Life*. Pennsylvania: Watch Tower Bible and Tract Society.

Watch Tower (1996) *Jehovah's Witnesses: Religious and Ethical Position on Medical Therapy, Child Care and Related Matters*. London: Hospital Information Service (Britain), Watch Tower.

Weller, P. (1997) *Religions in the UK: A Multifaith Directory*, 2nd edn. University of Derby in association with the Interfaith Network UK.

Internet resources

ChurchNet UK

http://www.churchnet.org.uk/

10.4 Hinduism

Traditions and beliefs

Hinduism refers to the religion of the population of India, although it is now practised worldwide. Hinduism is an ancient tradition and the term encompasses a variety of different schools of thought, beliefs and practices. It has been described as a way of life rather than a religion. There are an estimated 806 million Hindus worldwide and half a million in Britain (Weller 1997). There are approximately 160 Hindu places of worship in the United Kingdom.

Hindus believe in the existence of one supreme god but believe that the divine god takes many forms or demigods (*devas*). The most commonly worshipped of this is Vishnu who appeared on earth as Krishna or Rama. There are a variety of lesser gods.

Hindu scriptures are known as the Vedas and the most revered of these is the Bhagavad-Gita. Hindus believe in reincarnation. This cycle of birth and death is known as *Samsara*. The law of Karma states that all actions will reap certain reactions, good or bad depending on the action. The actions of a person will therefore determine both their fortunes in this life and the fate of their soul in the next life. The ultimate aim of Hindu religious life is to escape the cycle of birth and death (*Samsara*) and achieve union with Brahman (the supreme god). This attainment is described as *Moksha*. Because of its ancient origins and wide geographical spread, there are many differences of doctrine and practice within the Hindu tradition. The authority of the Vedas is however, generally accepted. In the United Kingdom, there are a variety of Hindu spiritual traditions (*Sampradaya*). Some have a strong Western presence, such as the International society of Krishna Consciousness.

Daily living, health and healing

The core values of Hinduism include respect for parents and elders, reverence for teachers, regard for guests, a general appreciation of the sanctity of life and *ahimsa* (non-violence). The cow is considered sacred (Weller 1997).

Hindu society is organized into *varnas* or castes. Individuals may only associate with members of their own *varna*. The four *varnas* are;

- Brahmins
- Kshatriyas
- Vaishyas
- Sudras

Within each *varna* an individual may belong to a subcaste or *jati*. The significance of *varnas* and *jati* varies according to the ethnic origin and individual beliefs of different Hindu families but is of particularly strong significance in Gujeratis. Sometimes individual Hindus may not wish to associate with members of different *varna*. Occasionally caste differences may cause difficulties between patients and health care staff. There are also Hindus who fall outside the traditional caste system, who have been described as *'untouchables'*.

As Hindus believe in non- violence (*ahimsa*) they are normally vegetarian and those who are not are required to abstain from beef. This includes any drugs derived from beef products. Vegetarianism generally precludes eating meat, fish and eggs or any products from slaughtered animals such as gelatine, animal fat and rennet. Some capsules and other medicines may contain gelatine and may be unacceptable. Hindus may also refrain from eating onions and garlic. Intoxicating drugs such as alcohol are normally refused and that may also extend to tea and coffee. Milk products are acceptable.

Many Hindus may wish to offer their food to a deity before eating and some may wish to fast at certain times of the year.

Hindus usually have strict differences in gender roles and female modesty is considered important. Hindu women strongly prefer to be treated by female medical and nursing staff. Hindus have strict standards of personal hygiene and prefer to wash in running water. Showers are preferable to baths and water should always be offered after giving a patient a bedpan. Patients should be given a jug of water and a wash bowl to enable them to wash their hands in running water (Green and Green 1992; Sullivan 1989).

Death and dying

There may be a variety of rituals performed at the end of life and after death. Hindus may appreciate assistance in contacting a local Hindu priest and the patient's family will wish to remain at the bedside. The priest or family may wish to read to the patient from Hindu scriptures and the family may prefer a single room at this time. The family may wish to bring money and gifts to be blessed by the dying patient and distributed to the poor.

After death the relatives may wish to carry out or assist in Last Offices and may wish the patient to be dressed in his or her own clothes. Relatives should be consulted as to their wishes in this respect before the body is handled. Some Hindus will be distressed if the body is handled by non-Hindus or members of the opposite sex. Any religious emblem such as a thread around the neck or wrist should *not* be removed from the body.

If no relatives are present the nurse should carry out the following procedure: wearing disposable gloves and apron the nurse should close the eyes and close the jaw, supporting it with a pillow if necessary. The body should be straightened. The body should *not* be washed.

If removal from the ward is necessary the body should be labelled and wrapped in a sheet. The patients should be left in his or her own clothing.

The patient should be cremated as soon as possible after death. Post mortem examination is accepted if legally necessary, but is otherwise refused. If post mortem examination takes place care must be taken that the body is sutured effectively with good cosmetic effect as the body will be washed by the family after the post mortem has taken place (Green and Green 1992; Sullivan 1989).

National contacts

National Council of Hindu Temples
c/o Shree Sanatan Mandir
Weymouth Street
off Catherine Street
Leicester. LE4 6FP
Telephone: 0116 266 1402

Hindu Council of the UK
c/o 150 Penn Road
Wolverhampton
West Midlands. WV3 0EN
Telephone: 01902 334 331

ISKCON Educational Services
Dharam Marg
Hillfield Lane
Aldenham
Watford
Herts. WD2 8EZ
Telephone: 01923 859 578

Local contacts (for personal use)

References and further reading

Bhaduri, R. (1984) 'Approach to loss and grief: a Hindu perspective', *Bereavement Care* 3(3): Taken from *Best of Bereavement Care*, No. 6 available from Cruse.

Black, J. (1991) 'Death and bereavement: the customs of Hindus, Sikhs and Moslems', *Bereavement Care* 10(1): 68.

Flood, G. (1996) *An Introduction to Hinduism*. Cambridge: Cambridge University Press.

Ghandial, H. (1983) 'Grieving Hindus in Britain', *Bereavement Care* 2(3): Taken from *Best of Bereavement Care*, No. 6 available from Cruse.

Green, J. and Green, M. (1992) *Dealing with Death: Practices and Procedures*. London: Chapman and Hall.

Keene, M. (1993) *Seekers after Truth: Hinduism, Buddhism, Sikhism*. Cambridge: Cambridge University Press.

Sullivan, L.E. (1989) *Healing and Restoring: Health and Medicine in the World's Religious Traditions*. New York: Macmillan.

Weller, P. (ed.) (1997) *Religions in the UK: A Multifaith Directory*. University of Derby in association with the Interfaith Network UK.

Internet resources

http: //www3.zdnet.com/yil/content/growth/philo/hindl.html

A guide to Hindu internet sites.

10.5 Islam

Traditions and beliefs

Muslims believe that the prophet Muhammad was the last and most important prophet from God (Allah) who completed the succession of prophets and their teachings. Abraham, Moses and Jesus are seen as the greatest of these prophets prior to Muhammad. Muhammad received revelations from the angel Gibreel (Gabriel) over a period of 23 years. These revelations form the bases of Islamic scripture, the holy Qur'an (Koran). Muhammad was born in the city of Makka (Mecca) which has now become a place of veneration and pilgrimage for Muslims.

Muslims must live according to Islamic Shari'ah (law). The five essential pillars of Islamic worship are:

1 *Shahadah* – the Islamic declaration of faith: *'la, ilaha illa-Llah, Muhammadon rasulu-Llah'* (There is no God except Allah, Muhammad is the messenger of Allah).
2 *Salat* – the ritual prayer five times a day. The times of these prayers vary throughout the year and prayer timetables are usually published by mosques. Prayers are obligatory from puberty onwards except for women who are menstruating or in the postnatal period or individuals who are not fully conscious. Ritual washing *must* take place prior to all prayers. During prayers the worshippers must face Makka. Prayer mats are available within the hospital should patients require them. Makka is in a south-easterly direction. A map of the hospital marked with the points of the compass is a useful aid.
3 *Zakat* – giving of alms to the needy.
4 *Ramadan* is a one-month period of prayer and fasting which occurs in the ninth month of the lunar year. Fasting must take place between sunrise and sunset. Children, the elderly, sick and pregnant are exempted from fasting during Ramadan. People who are exempted through illness may compensate by fasting for an equivalent period at another time of the year. Women who are menstruating must not fast.
5 *Hajj* pilgrimage to Makka at least once during an individual's lifetime (Weller 1997; Haneef 1979).

Approximately one-fifth of the world's population are Muslim. There are many different traditions and schools of thought in Islam. The two major traditions are Sunni Muslims (90 per cent of Muslims) and Shia Muslims (10 per cent). Within each of these two traditions there are divisions into different schools of thought. Muslim patients may therefore vary in their beliefs and in their adherence to Islamic laws. Local mosques and Muslim groups may, in addition, be organized according to the national origins of their members. There is also a mystical Islamic tradition known as Sufism. There are approximately 1–1.5 million Muslims in Britain (Weller 1997).

Daily living, health and healing

The Shari'ah governs all aspects of Muslim life, for example diet, personal hygiene and relations between men and women.

Food laws are important in Islam. The consumption of pork and any pork derivatives (including drugs etc.) is forbidden. Alcohol is also forbidden. All sea animals that do not have scales are also forbidden (i.e. shellfish).

Meat must be slaughtered according to Islamic law; it is then known as Halal meat. It is considered permissible by some Sunni Muslims to eat Kosher meat if Halal meat is not available, although this is not acceptable for Shia Muslims. If Halal meat is not available a vegetarian meal should be offered.

During the month of Ramadan Muslims should fast between sunrise and sunset. Most hospital patients will be exempt from this requirement. Medical and nursing staff should be aware that some Muslims will 'compensate' by an equivalent period of fasting, later in the year and may need advice as to whether this is medically advisable.

Personal hygiene is of great importance. Ritual washing of hands, face, mouth, nose, arms and feet must take place before prayer. Fresh running water is needed for washing and therefore showering facilities are required. Water is needed to wash down after urination and defecation. The left hand is used for washing and is therefore considered unclean and is not used when handling food etc. Menstruating women must wash the entire body after menstruation.

Women are often required to restrict their physical contact with men outside their family and to maintain strict public modesty. This may involve wearing a veil or head covering in public. Muslim women usually prefer not to be examined by male doctors. It is important to maintain privacy and modesty for Muslim women in hospital at all times. Male Muslim patients may also prefer to be cared for by staff of their own sex (IQRA Trust 1989).

Death and dying

Muslims believe in heaven and hell and believe that Allah will judge them for their actions on the Last Day or Judgement.

They believe that the circumstances of their death can be of significance to their afterlife. In particular, the dying Muslim should be mentally prepared for death and his or her last words should be the Shahadah (declaration of faith).

Relatives will want to read verses from the Qur'an (Koran) and pray for the patient's departing soul. Opportunities for quiet prayer will be appreciated, and in the terminal phase of illness patients may wish to be protected from the sounds of television, radio etc. If no relatives are available a member of the local Mosque should be contacted.

A dying patient should be turned to face Makka. If possible, the patient should be turned on their right side facing south-east). If this is not possible the patient may be placed on their back with their feet in a South Easterly direction and their head slightly raised (Amana 1994).

When the patient has died recitation of the Qur'an ceases. Immediately after death many relatives will want to carry out the following procedures:

- Close the eyes of the deceased.
- Bind the lower jaw with a cloth.
- Place an object on the abdomen to prevent it becoming inflated.
- Flex the joints of the arms and legs to stop them becoming rigid.
- Straighten the body and place the hands at the side of the body. It is not permitted to fold the arms across the chest.

At all times the body must be modestly covered with a clean sheet. If no relative or member of the local community is present, relatives may appreciate nursing staff carrying out the above procedure. Disposable gloves should be worn and the body should be handled by a member of staff of the same sex (Amana 1994).

The body should be handed over to the family or Muslim community as soon as possible and they will arrange washing, shrouding and burial according to Islamic law. In the case of patients dying of infectious diseases, relatives must be warned of the risks involved in washing the body.

Cremation is forbidden. Burial is normally within 24 hours. The family will appreciate release of the body as soon as is practicable. This may entail completing the necessary formalities for the release of a body outside of office hours. All staff should be familiar with the local procedure for releasing a body 'out of hours' to avoid confusion or delay. In some areas, the Registrar's office will arrange to open on Sundays and Bank Holidays to allow for registration of death where speedy burial is required for religious reasons. The All Muslim Funeral Society may be able to help with funeral expenses in cases of hardship.

Following amputation of any part of the body such as a limb, the patient should be consulted about disposal. Incineration of body parts should not be carried out without the express permission of the patient. Many Muslims will consider this as forbidden under Islamic law.

Until recently organ donation was usually regarded as contrary to Islamic law. However, in 1995 The Muslim Law Council issued a *fatwa* (religious ruling) permitting Muslims to donate organs (Muslim Law Council 1996). Trading in organs is prohibited. Some individual Muslims remain opposed to organ donation.

A post mortem examination should not be carried out unless it is legally necessary. Muslims regard post mortems as a desecration of the body. They may wish to discuss the details of a post mortem with the Coroner's office. During post mortem examination the corpse should be modestly covered. Relatives will appreciate a limited post mortem if at all possible. It will also be appreciated if the post mortem is carried out as speedily as possible.There is an on-call service of Coroner's officers who should be available out of hours via the local police station. Following post mortem examination, the organs must be replaced in their former positions. In particular, the contents of the skull should not be placed in the abdomen. Attention should be paid to suturing the corpse with good cosmetic effect, bearing in mind the fact that the body may be washed and shrouded by close relatives.

Following death shaving, cutting hair or trimming nails is not permitted. Photography of the corpse is not permitted.

National contacts

Information

Amana
PO Box 2842
London. W6 9ZH
Telephone: 0208 748 2424

IQRA Trust
24 Culross Street
London. W1Y 3HA
Telephone: 0207 491 1572

Islamic Centre England
140 Maida Vale
London. W9 1QB
Telephone: 0207 258 0526

Sufi Movement UK
Arama
Hawthorn Road
Highfield
Southampton
Hampshire. SO17 1PX
Telephone: 02380 558 357

Welfare organizations

All Muslim Funeral Society
127 Kingsway
Luton
Bedfordshire. LU1 1TS
Telephone: 01582 451 853

British Muslim Association
58 Parkway
West Wimbledon
London. SW20 9HF
Telephone: 0208 542 8507

Muslim Women's Helpline
Room 7, 11 Main Drive
East Lane Estate
Wembley
Middlesex. HA8 7NA
Telephone: 0208 908 3205

Local contacts (for personal use)

References and further reading

Amana (1994) Muslim Patients (mimeo).
Black, J. (1991) 'Death and bereavement: the customs of Hindus, Sikhs and Mulims', *Bereavement Care* 10(1): 68.
Gatrad, A. (1994) 'Muslim customs surrounding death, bereavement, postmortem examinations and organ transplant', *British Medical Journal* 309: 521–3.
Hakimul Ummat Mavlana Ashraf Ali (Undated) *Bahishti Zewar: Requisites of Islam*. Delhi: Dini Book Depot.
Haneef, S. (1979) *What Everyone Should Know about Islam and Muslims*. Lahore: Kazi Publications.
Henley, A. (1982) *Caring for Muslims and Their Families: Religious Aspects of Care*. Cambridge: National Extension College.
IQRA Trust (1988) *Local Authority Facilities for Muslim Burial*. Research Report No. 3.
IQRA Trust (1989) *National Health Service Hospital Facilities for Muslim Patients*. Research Report No. 4.
Muslim Law (Shari'ah) Council (1996) 'The Muslim Law (Shari'ah) Council and organ transplants', *Accident and Emergency Nursing* 4(?): 73–5.
Muslim World League (undated) *Funeral Regulations in Islam*.
Rispler-Chain, V. (1993) 'The ethics of post mortem examinations in contemporary Islam', *Journal of Medical Ethics* 19: 164–8.
Sheikh, A. (1998) 'Death and dying: a Muslim perspective', *Journal of the Royal Society of Medicine* 91(3): 138–40.
Sullivan, L. (1989) *Healing and Restoring: Health and Medicine in the World's Religious Traditions*. New York: Macmillan.
Weller, P. (1997) *Religions in the UK: A Multifaith Directory*, 2nd edn. University of Derby in association with the Interfaith Network UK.

Internet resources

The website of the IQRA trust
http://www.iqra.org.uk

10.6 Jainism

Traditions and beliefs

Jainism was founded in India in the sixth century BC. Jains follow the teaching of twenty-four religious teachers known as Jinas or Tirthankaras (ford makers). Their words are laid down in a number of Jain scriptures (*Shruta*). Jains believe in *Samsara* (the cycle of birth, death and reincarnation) and believe that the only way to escape from this cycle is through achieving spiritual perfection (*Moksha* or *Nirvana*).

Jains seek to live according to the Three Jewels: right faith, right knowledge and right conduct. There are five *Vratas* (vows) governing conduct. These are *ahimsa* (non- injury to all living creatures), *satya* (truthfulness), *asteya* (not stealing), *brachmacharya* (chastity) and *aparigrahi* (non-materialism). Lay people follow these rules with less strictness than Jain monks, i.e. for lay Jains chastity means faithfulness and for Jain monks it means complete celibacy.

There are two main groups of Jain monks, the Shretambaras (white robed monks) and Digambaras (sky clad monks). The majority of Jains in this country are Shretambaras. Most Jains in this country are Gujerati in origin. Jain social groupings may be further subdivided according to the caste origins of their members. There are approximately 30,000 Jains in the UK (Weller 1997).

Daily living, health and healing

The principle of *ahimsa* means that Jains are strict vegetarians or vegans and may also refrain from root vegetables, honey and alcohol. Some Jains may also refrain from eating between sunrise and sunset. Jains may wish to offer worship (*puja*) three times a day.

Jains will appreciate assistance in maintaining strict standards of hygiene and may appreciate the use of running water for washing.

Death and dying

Jains believe that the last moment of life has an influence on an individual's next life. Jains may therefore wish assistance in religious observances at the end of life. Some Jains may be unhappy to take drugs that affect their mental clarity. It is important to discuss the effects of drugs with Jain patients. Early Jain monks believed that if illness or old age prevented a monk from performing his religious duties then he should fast until he achieved a religious death (*sallekhana*). *Sallekhana* is rarely practised today, although it still has an influence on the Jain attitude to death.

After death, relatives should be consulted concerning rites after death and especially before the commencement of Last Offices. If no relatives are immediately available the nurses should proceed with limited laying out, as for a Hindu patient (see above). The organizations listed below can be contacted for further advice and information.

National contacts

Institute of Jainology
Unit 18, Silicon Business Centre
26–28 Wandsworth Road
Greenford
Middlesex. UB6 7JZ

Jain Academy
20 St James Close
London. NW11 9QX
Telephone: 0208 455 5573

Local contacts (for personal use)

References and further reading

Dundas, P. (1992) *The Jains*. London: Routledge.
New Encyclopedia Britannica (1989) 15th edn. 'Jainism'. Chicago: Encyclopedia Britannica.
Sampson, C. (1982) *The Neglected Ethic*. London: McGraw Hill.
Smart, Ninian (1992) *The World's Religions*. Cambridge: Cambridge University Press.
Weller, P. (ed.) (1993) *Religions in the UK: A Multifaith Directory*. University of Derby in
  association with the Interfaith Network UK.

Internet resources

http: //www.cs.colostate.edu/n/nalaiya/hainhlinks.html.
A guide to Jain websites.

10.7 Judaism

Traditions and beliefs

Judaism is the religion of the Jewish people. The Jewish population of the
UK is estimated at approximately 300,000. Jews believe in one God who
created the universe. The main Jewish scriptures are the Torah and
Talmud, which lay down the rules for daily life and worship. The main
precepts of Judaism are to worship one God and to obey the Ten
Commandments.

The Jewish community in this country is comprised mainly of
Ashkenazi Jews who migrated here from Central and Eastern Europe.

Although most Jews in this country today speak English some Ashkenazi Jews speak a Judaeo-German dialect known as Yiddish. There is a small community of Sephardi Jews who are Spanish in origin and whose original language, Ladino, was Spanish in origin. Hebrew is the language of the Bible and most Jewish people learn it as children at synagogue (Weller 1997).

Jewish communities cover a wide spectrum of religious observance. Some belong to orthodox or ultra-orthodox (Chasidic) communities. Others belong to liberal progressive or reform communities. These different Jewish traditions observe Jewish law with variable strictness. The Jewish patient in hospital will have different requirements depending on the tradition he or she belongs to.

Key Jewish traditions include observance of the Sabbath (Shabbat) and Jewish food regulations.

The Sabbath is central to Jewish life. It is celebrated on Saturday as a day of rest and worship. The Sabbath begins half an hour before sunset on Friday night and finishes at sunset on Saturday. Religious ceremonies take place both at home and at synagogue during the Sabbath. Jews are forbidden to work on the Sabbath; this is interpreted with varying degrees of strictness depending on the particular Jewish tradition. The Jewish duty to save lives always takes precedence over observance of the Sabbath.

Jewish dietary law states that meat can only be consumed from animals with cloven hooves which chew the cud, such as cows, sheep and goats. Meat must be ritually slaughtered and is described as Kosher meat. Pig and rabbit is not acceptable, although birds such as chicken are considered an acceptable food.

Fish must have fins and scales, so eating shellfish is not permitted. Jewish law also prohibits mixing meat and milk products (Weller 1997).

There are a number of important ceremonies in Jewish life. In particular most people will be familiar with the circumcision of males on the eighth day of life. On occasions, Jewish families may seek medical advice about this ceremony or may request that it is carried out in hospital rather than by the local Mohel (trained circumciser). Medical attitudes vary regarding circumcision for religious reasons.

At 13 years of age Jewish boys undertake the ceremony of Barmitzvah. This involves reading the weekly portion of the Torah in Hebrew, usually at the Sabbath Service in the synagogue. The Barmitzvah symbolizes that the boy has come of age and can assume a place in the adult Jewish religious community. In liberal and progressive Judaism, there is an equivalent ceremony for Jewish girls called the Batmitzvah.

Daily living, health and healing

All Jewish patients will wish to avoid pork and pork products and also shellfish. Many Jewish patients will wish to eat only ritually prepared 'Kosher' food. If Kosher food is not available a vegetarian diet may be acceptable.

Many Jewish patients observe strict rules regarding the Sabbath and Orthodox patients may not be permitted to travel, make phone calls etc.

between sunset on Friday and nightfall on Saturday. Nurses should be mindful of this when making discharge arrangements.

Orthodox Jewish women may wish to keep their head and body covered in public and their modesty and privacy should be maintained. Jewish patients may also require facilities for daily prayers.

Jews believe strongly in the sanctity of life and often hold the medical professions in high esteem (Neuberger 1994).

Death and dying

There are two basic principles governing Jewish traditions surrounding death. The first is *'kavod hamet'*, the requirement to honour the dead. The second is *'nichen avelin'*, the requirement to comfort mourners.

If a Jewish patient is approaching death, the next of kin should be contacted. If no relatives are available, the Jewish chaplain or a member of the patient's synagogue should be contacted. The rituals performed as death approaches allow the family time to say farewell to the patient. A dying person should not be left alone and the dying Jew may wish to hear or recite prayers. In the Orthodox tradition there will be a rite of 'confession' in which the dying person asks forgiveness for past errors. Care of the patient following death will vary according to the tradition from which the patient comes. If the advice of the patient's family is not available the guidelines below can be followed. They will apply to most Orthodox Jews and some from other traditions.

- Following death the body should remain untouched for 20 minutes. If after this period no member of the family or Jewish community is available, the following procedure should be carried out by nursing staff:
- The eyes and mouth should be closed. The jaw should be closed and held in place by a bandage tied above the head.
- The fingers of each hand should be straightened and the arms placed at the side of the body. Feet and legs should be straightened.
- Tubes or lines such as drains, IV lines etc. should be removed and any incisions covered except in cases where these must be retained for Coroner's enquiries (see Chapter 8).
- Excess dirt, such as blood, urine, faeces or vomit, should be wiped away. The body should not, however, be washed.
- The patient should remain in the clothes in which she/he died and the body should not be shrouded.
- The body should be wrapped in a sheet and if relatives are still unavailable it can be transported to the hospital mortuary until arrangements are made for the family to take over responsibility for the body. In most areas with a Jewish community there is a Jewish burial society who will superintend the care of deceased Jews.

During the Jewish Sabbath it will not be possible to arrange for removal of the body or for attendance on the body and it should remain in the mortuary until after the Sabbath.

Washing and preparing the body for burial are carried out by the Jewish community. The body should be handled as little as possible by hospital staff and disposable gloves may be worn. Jewish family members should be advised of any dangers in attending to the deceased in cases of infectious disease. It is helpful if the documentation accompanying the deceased is labelled with the word Jewish. Writing on the body itself should not occur; it is considered offensive.

Jewish law requires that the body remains intact after death and post mortem examination is regarded as a desecration. Relatives may be upset by a request for post mortem examination where this is not required by law. Jewish law forbids cremation and requires that the body is buried as soon as possible after death. The relatives will therefore require assistance in arranging speedy release of the body and this may require 'out of hours' arrangements. These arrangements should be clearly understood by all staff.

If a Coroner's post mortem is required the Coroner's officer should be contacted to expedite arrangements. There is an on-call service of Coroner's officers who should be available out of hours via the local police station. In some areas, the Registrar's office will arrange to open on Sundays and Bank Holidays to allow for registration of death where speedy burial is required for religious reasons. The Jewish Burial Society should know whether this service is offered in the local area.

Following stillbirths, burial is required and in the event of miscarriage many Jewish parents will also wish to arrange for the funeral of the fetus.

The tradition of *kavod hamet* means that many Jewish people believe that a body should not be left unattended after death and prior to burial Jewish relatives may therefore require facilities to remain with the deceased, either at the bedside or in the mortuary. Facilities should be made available to relatives wishing to watch the body.

The tradition of *nichen avelin* means that the bereaved go through a formal period of mourning during which they receive much support from their community.

Traditions surrounding death will, of course, vary between individual members of different Jewish traditions. For example, many modern non-Orthodox Jews will now accept cremation. In the absence of knowledge of the precise beliefs of the individual, it is probably best to err on the side of caution until further information is obtained.

Organ donation is not expressly forbidden, although opinions may vary and some Jews may have religious objections to this practice.

National contacts

Information

> **Office of the Chief Rabbi (Orthodox)**
> 735 High Road
> North Finchley
> London. WC1N 9HN
> Telephone: 0208 343 6301

Union of Liberal and Progressive Synagogues
The Montagu Centre
21 Maple Street
London. W1P 6DS
Telephone: 0207 580 1663

Reform Synagogues of Great Britain
The Sternberg Centre for Judaism
80 East End Road
Finchley
London. N3 2SY
Telephone: 0208 349 4731

Scottish Council of Synagogues
28 Field Road
Busby
Glasgow
Strathclyde. G76 8SE
Telephone: 0141 644 3411

Welfare organizations

Jewish AIDS Trust
HIV Education Unit
Colindale Hospital
Colindale Avenue
London. NW9 5HG
Telephone: 0208 200 0369

Jewish Bereavement Counselling Service
PO Box 6748
London. N3 3BX
Telephone: 0208 349 0839

Jewish Care
Stuart Young House
221 Golders Green Road
London. NW1 9DQ
Telephone: 0208 458 3282

Jewish Care Scotland
May Terrace
Giffnock
Glasgow
Strathclyde. G46 6LD
Telephone: 0141 620 1800

Jewish Crisis Helpline (Miyad)
23 Ravenshurst Avenue
Hendon
London. NW4 4EE
Telephone: 0208 203 6311

League of Jewish Women
24–32 Stephenson Way
London. NW1 2JW
Telephone: 0207 387 7688

Local contacts (for personal use)

References and further reading

Irish, D.(1990) *Ethnic Variations in Dying, Death and Grief.* Washington: Taylor and Francis.
Katz, J.S. (1996) 'Caring for Jewish people in a multicultural religious society', *International Journal of Palliative Nursing* 2(1): 43–7.
Manchester Beth Din (1992) *Guidelines for Dealing with Dying and Deceased Jewish Patients.* Manchester: Manchester Beth Din.
Neuberger, J. (1994) 'A Jewish perspective on palliative care', *Palliative Care Today* 3(3): 32–3.
Rabinowicz, H. (1979) 'The Jewish view of death', *Nursing Times* May 3: 757.
Stenberg, H. (1984) 'Jewish mourning practices: do they help?', *Bereavement Care* 3(2): Taken from the *Best of Bereavement Care*, No. 6 available from Cruse.
Sullivan, L. (ed.) (1989) *Healing and Restoring: Health and Medicine in the World's Religious Traditions.* New York: Macmillan.
Weller, P. (1997) *Religions in the UK: A Multifaith Directory*, 2nd edn. University of Derby in association with the Interfaith Network UK.

Internet resources

http: //www.shemayisrael.co.il/burial/needs.htm

An Orthodox Israeli site discussing the religious needs of Orthodox patients.

10.8 The Sikh faith

Traditions and beliefs

The Sikh religion is founded on the teachings of ten Gurus. The first of these Gurus and the founder of Sikhism was Guru Nanak Dev Ji (1469–1539). Guru Nanak was born in Talwandi in the Punjab (now in Pakistan) and in his adult life he travelled extensively through Asia as a preacher. He preached universal love and stressed the virtues of truthfulness, kindness, generosity and the equality of men. He was opposed to superstition and ritual and preached the one-ness of God. He eventually settled at Kartapur in Punjab and founded the Sikh community His teachings were followed by nine more Sikh gurus in the next 239 years. These

Gurus are believed to convey God's word. Following the death of the tenth Guru, Gobind Singh Ji, religious authority was vested in Sikh scriptures.

Guru Gobind Singh Ji instituted the ceremony of Amrit Pahul. In this ceremony Sikhs pledge their allegiance to their religion and as a symbol of this they undertake to wear the 5 'K's:

- *Kesh* (uncut hair usually worn in a turban).
- *Kangha* (a small comb worn in the hair).
- *Kara* (the steel bangle, a reminder to do good).
- *Kachhahera* (a knee length garment (like shorts) symbolizing modesty and restraint).
- *Kirpan* (a short sword symbolizing dignity and self respect).
- Male Sikhs take the name Singh (lion) and females the name Kaur (princess). This practice originated to emphasize Sikh belief in equality and opposition to the caste system.

Daily living, health and healing

Sikhs are required to abstain from alcohol, tobacco and drugs. Sikhs are prohibited from eating beef and may also abstain from eating pork. Some Sikhs will be vegetarian or vegan. Sikhs are expected to rise early and to say morning prayers following a bath or shower. Evening prayers are recited before retiring to bed. A quiet area of the ward may be appreciated for prayers.

Sikhs will often prefer to shower rather than bath and will be grateful for washing facilities before meals and after using a bedpan or urinal. Sikh women may prefer to be examined by a female doctor. A Sikh man should not be required to remove any of the 5 Ks unless strictly necessary. If it is necessary for a Sikh to be shaved or have hair cut, the reasons for this should be carefully explained and permission obtained. In general, the five 'Ks' should not be removed or disturbed by health care staff without permission.

Death and dying

A dying Sikh may wish to recite prayers or read passages from the Sikh scriptures. If he or she is too ill to do so, a relative or member of the Sikh community may do so instead. Staff should ask patients and relatives if they have any special requirements.

Following a death some relatives may wish to carry out Last Offices. There is no religious prohibition against health care staff handling the body but relatives should be consulted. The Five 'K's *must* be respected.

The majority of Sikhs would prefer to avoid post mortem examination unless it is legally required. Organ donation is permitted, but some Sikhs may have misgivings about mutilation of the body (Exley 1996).

At death Sikhs normally cremate the body, and cremation should take place as soon as possible, preferably within 24 hours. It is unlikely, however, that a local crematorium will be able to arrange cremation at such short notice and a wait of a few days is usual. It should be noted that a body *must not* be released for cremation if there is any likelihood that it will be referred to the Coroner. It is not normal practice to release a body for cremation 'out of hours.'

National contacts

Sikh Missionary Society UK
10 Featherstone Road
Southall
Middlesex. UB2 5AA
Telephone: 0208 574 1902

Sikh Educational and Cultural Association (UK)
Sat Nam Kutia
18 Farmcroft
Gravesend
Kent. DA11 7LT
Telephone: 01474 332356

World Sikh Foundation
88 Mollison Way
Edgware
Middlesex. HA8 5QW
Telephone: 0208 952 1215

Local contacts (for personal use)

References and further reading

Black, J. (1991) 'Death and bereavement: the customs of Hindus, Sikhs and Muslims', *Bereavement Care* 10(1): 6–8.

Cole, W.O. and Sambhi, P. (1995) *The Sikhs, Their Religious Beliefs and Practices*. London: Sussex Academic Press.

Exley, C. (1996) 'Attitudes and beliefs within the Sikh community regarding organ donation: a pilot study', *Social Science and Medicine* 43(1): 23–8.

Hinnells, J. (1996) *A New Handbook of Living Religions*. Oxford: Blackwells.

Sindhu, G.S. (1988) *The Sikh Temple*. Southall: Sikh Missionary Society.

Singh, K.S. (1994) *Sikh Patients in Hospital*. Birmingham: Sikh Educational and Cultural Association.

Weller, P. (1997) *Religions in the UK: A Multifaith Directory*. University of Derby in Association with the Interfaith Network UK.

Internet resources

The Sikhism home page produced by Sandeep Singh Brar

http: //www.sikhs.org/rehit.htm

10.9 The Zoroastrian faith

Traditions and beliefs

Zoroastrianism is the religion of the followers of the prophet Zoroaster (Zarethustra). Zoroaster is believed to have lived in Iran some time between 6000 BC and 1700 BC. Zoroastrians believe in a supreme God Ahura Mazda, who is the source of *asha* (truth, righteousness, order and justice). Zoroastrians also believe in the existence of a destructive spirit, Angra Maingo, which is responsible for misery, suffering, disorder and death. Zoroastrians believe that humans must oppose the evil Angra Maingo through good thoughts, good words and good deeds.

Zoroastrians believe that Ahura Mazda created both the spiritual and material worlds and humans have a duty to care for both. They believe therefore in being active in promoting good in society and in caring for the Earth. Zoroastrians therefore have a highly developed moral code. Zoroastrian beliefs have had a major impact on other world religions, especially Christianity. As a result of religious persecution the Zoroastrian community has become dispersed throughout the world. There is a major Zoroastrian community in India, where they are known as Parsees (Persian). There are several thousand Zoroastrians living in Britain, many of whom are Parsee in origin. As with other major world religions there are liberal and orthodox branches of the Zoroastrian faith and so individual patients may vary in the extent to which they observe Zoroastrian rituals and practices.

Daily living, health and healing

Zoroastrian children are initiated into the faith between the ages of 7 and 11 in a ceremony known as the *navjote* (new birth). After this ceremony the child is invested with the garments the *sudreh* and the *kushti*, which are to be worn at all times. The *sudreh* is a white cotton or muslin shirt symbolizing purity and the *kushti* is a girdle woven of seventy-two strands of lambs' wood symbolizing the seventy two chapters of the Yasna (Liturgy). Special prayers are said during the construction of these garments and they are seen as a protection against evil. The patient will therefore wish to continue to wear these garments at all times in hospital.

For the purposes of prayer the day is divided into five times and the Zoroastrian patient may wish to offer prayers (*namah*) at these times. At prayer, Zoroastrians wash hands, face and feet and should turn towards the sun or artificial light if no natural light is available. The *kushti* is untied and held before them and retied after the completion of prayers. The Zoroastrian patient may require assistance with this whilst in hospital. In particular Zoroastrians will require assistance in maintaining their customary standards of cleanliness in hospital and will prefer running water to wash in. There are no Zoroastrian dietary laws but some Zoroastrians may refrain from pork or beef or be vegetarian.

Death and dying

The relatives of the dying patient have a duty to recite prayers to the patient. The patient, if conscious, is required to join in these prayers.

Zoroastrians believe that death is the separation of body and soul. On the fourth day after death, the soul is judged at the Chinuat Bridge (Bridge of the Separator). Here the soul's good words, deeds and thoughts are weighed against the evil ones. Then the soul either ascends to heaven (The Realm of Light) or descends to hell (The Realm of Darkness and Separation) (Weller 1997)

Zoroastrians believe that the human body becomes corrupted as soon as breath has left it. They believe therefore that the body should be disposed of as quickly as possible and will therefore wish for the funeral to take place as soon as possible after death. After death the body is washed and dressed in the *sudrah* and *kushti* and a long white robe and cap or scarf maybe placed over the *sudrah*. The hospital shroud may be considered suitable. Relatives should be consulted to find out their preferences and whether they wish to wash and dress the patient or would prefer nursing staff to do so. In some cases Zoroastrians will not wish the body to be touched by someone from outside the faith.

Post mortems are disliked and are likely to be refused by relatives if at all possible. Organ donation and blood transfusion are also disliked by orthodox Zoroastrians and are likely to be refused.

Zoroastrians believe that the corpse should not pollute earth, fire or water and therefore in areas where there is a large Zoroastrian community, i.e. in India, bodies are disposed of in a Tower of Silence (*dokhma*). This is a cylindrical building built in three concentric circles, one each for men, women and children, with a deep pit at the centre. Here the bodies are exposed on stone ledges to be consumed by vultures; the bones are afterwards swept into the pit to be destroyed by lime. Zoroastrians consider this method to be ecologically sound, but in Britain if bodies are not flown back to India for disposal they are buried at the Zoroastrian cemetery in Brookwood in Surrey which was established in 1863.

National contacts

Zoroastrian Trust Funds of Europe
88 Compagne Gardens
London. NW6 3RU
Telephone: 0207 328 6018

World Zoroastrian Organization
135 Tennison Road
South Norwood
London. SE25 5NF
Telephone: 01279 503771

Local contacts (for personal use)

References and further reading

Homji, H.B.M. (1989) *Zoroastrianism: Contemporary Perception of Ancient Wisdom*. Toronto: HBM Homji.
Nigosian, S.A. (1996) 'Tradition and modernity in contemporary Zoroastrian communities', *Journal of Asian and African Studies* 31: 206–16.
New Encyclopedia Britannica (1989) 15th edn. 'Zoroastrianism and Parsiism', Chicago: Encyclopedia Britannica 29: 1146–7.
Polson, C.J. and Marshall, T.K. (1975) *The Disposal of the Dead*. London: English University Press.
Taraporewala, I.J.S. (1965) *The Religion of Zarethustra*. Bombay: Bombay University Press.
Weller, P. (1993) *Religions in the UK: A Multifaith Directory*. University of Derby in association with the Interfaith Network UK.

10.10 New religious movements (cults)

The twentieth century witnessed an enormous growth in new religious movements (cults). The key features of these movements are that they are new, many prove to be short lived and their growth is thought to be a result of the rapid social change that is a feature of modern life.

Because new religious movements are new and all of their members are converts they tend to be more enthusiastic and fervent in their beliefs and practices than many members of established religions. Often new religious movements are founded by a charismatic leader who has great authority over the lives of the members of the movement. The extreme exercise of this authority by some leaders of new religious movements, such as the People's Temple in Jonestown and the Branch Davidians in Waco, have led to some public concern about new religious movements, or 'cults' as they are sometimes described. In fact, most new religious movements do not exercise this kind of extreme authority over their members; members choose to join them and they are generally benign in their effects (Barker 1989).

Some writers suggest that cult groups engage in coercion and '*brainwashing.*' (Singer 1992; West 1993). This has led to the growth of anti-cult groups who campaign against new religious movements and sometimes forcibly remove individuals from cults in order to *'deprogramme'* them. Some extreme anti-cult groups have been responsible for human rights abuses similar to those perpetrated by extreme cults themselves; this mentality may perhaps be explained by the involvement of ex-cult members in some anti-cult groups. Relatives of cult members should be warned against *'exit counsellors'* and *'deprogrammers'*, especially those who demand money for their services.

While the majority of members of new religious movements come to no harm as a result of their religious affiliation there are some groups which can pose a threat to the health and welfare of their members. Particular danger signals are a movement that cuts itself off from society, drawing sharp boundaries between 'them' and 'us' and a leader who claims divine authority over members. Other warning signals are when cult members allow important decisions over their lives to be made by others. This can, of course, be relevant in the health care setting (Barker 1989).

Young and Griffiths (1992) argue that the suggestion that cults can 'brainwash' individuals so that they are no longer in control of their thoughts is unconvincing. They point out, however, that cult members may be exposed to systematic misinformation and deception. They argue that it is more helpful to approach this issue as one of informed consent. This is of particular relevance when addressing the issue of informed consent and refusal of medical treatment. In particular, their arguments may have a special relevance for the consideration of advance directives refusing medical treatment on religious grounds.

It is not always easy to distinguish between people who have chosen to live their lives in a way that seems incomprehensible to us as outsiders and people who are under psychological duress. In general, we should assume that competent adults have made their own decisions and are responsible for them. In general, membership of a religious organization confers health benefits (Jarvis and Northcutt 1987). However, there is some evidence that membership of zealous religious groups can lead to psychiatric morbidity in some individuals (Kilger 1994).

In some cases new religious movements may be hostile to Western medicine or may encourage converts to engage in activities such as extreme fasting that can be damaging to physical health. For some new religious movements illness may be taken as a sign of weakness or sin and this can result in converts being unwilling or unable to seek appropriate medical treatment.

Where patients are refusing treatment for religious reasons medical and nursing staff should try to ensure that the patient is making his or her own decision and is competent to do so. This may mean ensuring that the patient is not exposed to psychological pressure from members of the religious group and it may be necessary to ask such members to leave for a time so that the patient has the space to make his or her own decision. It may also be important to ensure that members of the religious groups do not prevent family and friends who are outside the group from contacting the patient. In some cases legal advice may be needed (see also Chapter 4).

Staff may come into contact with the families of converts to new religious movements. In many cases families may be hurt and bewildered that their relative has joined a movement whose beliefs and practices may seem bizarre and unacceptable to them. The most important advice for families of converts is to keep in touch with the convert and to try to maintain a positive relationship, avoiding hostile criticism of the convert. An organization called *Inform* exists to disseminate unbiased information about new religious movements and can be contacted for advice. Inform is an information and advice organization and not a counselling organization. However, if enquirers are experiencing difficulties it can put them in touch with individuals or organizations who may be able to help.

National contacts

INFORM
(Information Network Focus on Religious Movements)
Houghton Street
London. WC2A 2AE
Telephone: 0207 955 7654

Cult Information Centre
BCM Cults
London. WC1N 3XX
Telephone: 0208 651 3322

Some examples of new religious movements

Church of Scientology

The Church of Scientology was founded in 1954 by L Ron Hubbard, a former science fiction writer. The basic philosophy of the movement is the use of 'dianetic therapy' in which an 'auditor' helps people to erase harmful influences called 'engrams' which have been imprinted in their mind in the past in this life or a previous incarnation. Successful 'auditing' leads to the person becoming 'clear' and they are then thought to achieve optimum functioning.

The movement has an aggressive and hostile stance towards psychiatry and has been involved in a number of organizations that have campaigned against orthodox psychiatry.

One of the main complaints against the organization has been the high cost of therapy and many clients of the organization have found themselves running up debts of thousands of pounds (Barker 1989). The movement is eager to make contact with individuals with mental health problems and such individuals may need to be warned of the possible costs of becoming involved with Scientology.

Paganism (occultism, witchcraft etc.)

The past hundred years has seen the revival of a number of pre-Christian beliefs and practices and this has led to the creation of a variety of neo-pagan groups. There are a diversity of new Pagan groups, including Druidry, Odinism, Shamanism and Witchcraft (Wicca). Pagans emphasize a close relationship with nature.

The Pagan Federation suggests that the Pagan ethic is 'Do what thou wilt, but harm none'. It is important to distinguish Paganism from Satanism; there is no belief in or worship of any 'devil' figure in Paganism. The diversity of Pagan and 'new age' beliefs and the lack of formal organizations associated with most of them means that individual patients will need to be asked how their needs can be satisfied in hospital and some Pagans may fear hostility and be reluctant to reveal their beliefs to outsiders.

National contacts

The Pagan Federation
BM Box 7097
London. WC1N 3XX
Telephone: 01691 671 066

The Pagan Hospice and Funeral Trust
BM Box 3337
London. WC1N 3XX

Internet resources

The Pagan Federation website
http: //sunacm.swan.ac.uk./paganfed/

Rastafarianism

Rastafarianism grew out of the 'back to Africa' movement started in Jamaica in the 1930s by Marcus Garvey. Rastafarians believe that Haile Selassie I, the Emperor of Ethiopia, (otherwise named Ras (Prince) Tafari, hence Rastafarianism) was a direct descendant of the biblical King David and was the modern Messiah. Rastafarians accept biblical teachings, and the teachings of the Old Testament are particularly important to them. They believe that God (Jah) created all men equal but especially favours blacks; they believe that they are the 'true Jews' and that their oppression in the white social system (Babylon) will eventually be ended with their return to Africa.

Rastafarians can be distinguished by their 'dreadlocks' and may also often wear the Rastafarian colours of red, black, green and gold. Rastafarians do not normally drink alcohol and are often vegetarian. Pork is normally prohibited. Some Rastafarians believe that smoking marijuana ('*ganga*') has religious significance. Some Rastafarians are hostile towards Western medicine and may prefer to use alternative therapies such as herbalism. Objection to blood transfusion is also common among Rastafarians. Post mortem examination would be distasteful to most Rastafarians.

There are few formal organizations associated with Rastafarians and individuals may vary in their adherence to its beliefs and tenets. It should also be remembered that 'dreadlocks' have become fashionable and do not always signify Rastafarian beliefs.

National contacts

The Rastafarian Society
290–296 Tottenham High Road
London. N15 4AJ
Telephone: 0208 808 2185

The Unification Church

The Unification Church was founded by Rev. Sun Myung Moon in Korea in 1954. The Church accepts the teachings of the Old and New Testaments supplemented with further revelations by Rev. Moon. The Church is particularly hostile to communism.

The Church runs a number of successful businesses and has become extremely wealthy worldwide. Its members are required to devote themselves to the organization and spend time fund raising for the organization under the guise of a number of 'charitable' enterprises. The church lost a libel suit against the *Daily Mail* which had accused it of brainwashing members and of breaking up families. However, in spite of such accusations its turnover of members is extremely high.

References and further reading

Barker, E. (1989) *New Religious Movements: A Practical Introduction*. London: HMSO.
Galanter, M. (1989) *Cults: Faith, Healing and Coercion*. Oxford: Oxford University Press.
Jarvis, G. and Northcutt, H. (1987) 'Religion and differences in morbidity and mortality', *Social Science and Medicine* 25(7): 813–24.
Kilger, R. (1994) 'Somatisation, social control and illness production in a religious cult', *Culture, Medicine and Psychiatry* 18(2): 215–45.
The Pagan Federation (1992) *The Pagan Federation Information Pack*, 2nd edn. London: Pagan Federation.
Singer, M. (1992) 'Cults, coercion and continuity', *Cultic Studies Journal* 19(2): 163–89.
Weller, P. (1997) *Religions in the UK: A Multifaith Directory*. University of Derby in association with the Interfaith Network UK.
West, L.J. (1993) 'A psychiatric overview of cult-related phenomena', *Journal of the American Academy of Psychoanalysis* 21(1): 1–19.
Young, J. and Griffiths, E. (1992) 'A critical evaluation of coercive persuasion as used in the assessment of cults', *Behavioural Sciences and the Law* 10: 89–101.

10.11 Humanism/atheism

It is important to be aware that patients without religious beliefs may still have spiritual beliefs if 'spirituality' is understood as a search for meaning in life.

Atheists deny the existence of God, having made a conscious decision to do so; agnostics, however, argue that it is impossible to prove or disprove God's existence and are therefore neither believers nor unbelievers. Humanists argue that there is no God and that individuals must therefore act for the benefit of all mankind. Some 'unbelievers' will not adhere to any of the above positions but will simply not have given thought to religious issues. Non-believers may feel embarrassed about being asked about their religious affiliation but may resent being recorded as 'Church of England' if this is not their belief.

Some atheist or humanist patients may wish to be assured that they can arrange a non-religious funeral. The British Humanist Association publish a useful booklet entitled *Funerals Without God*, giving detailed information on arranging secular funerals.

National contacts

British Humanist Association
14 Lamb's Conduit Passage
London. WC1R 4RH

Further reading

Burnard, P. (1988) 'The spiritual needs of atheists and agnostics', *Professional Nurse* December: 130–2.

Index